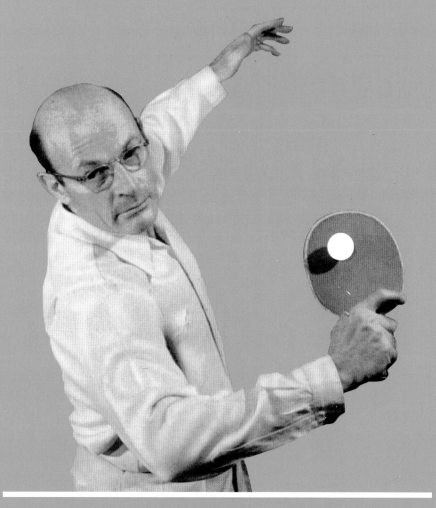

EVERYTHING YOU KNOW IS PONG

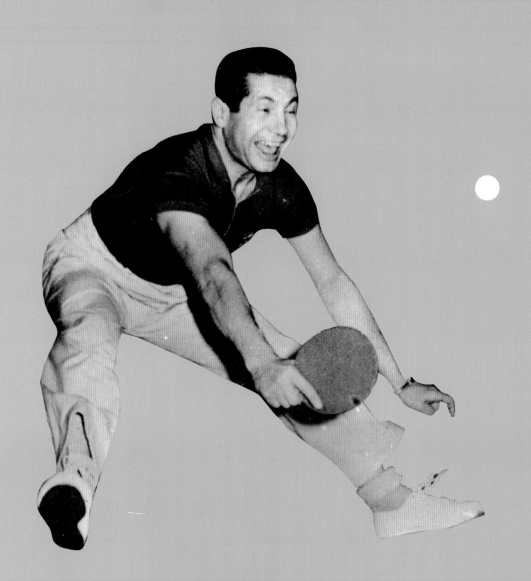

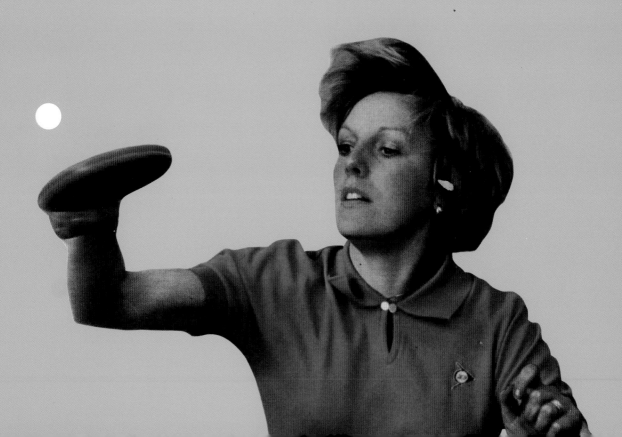

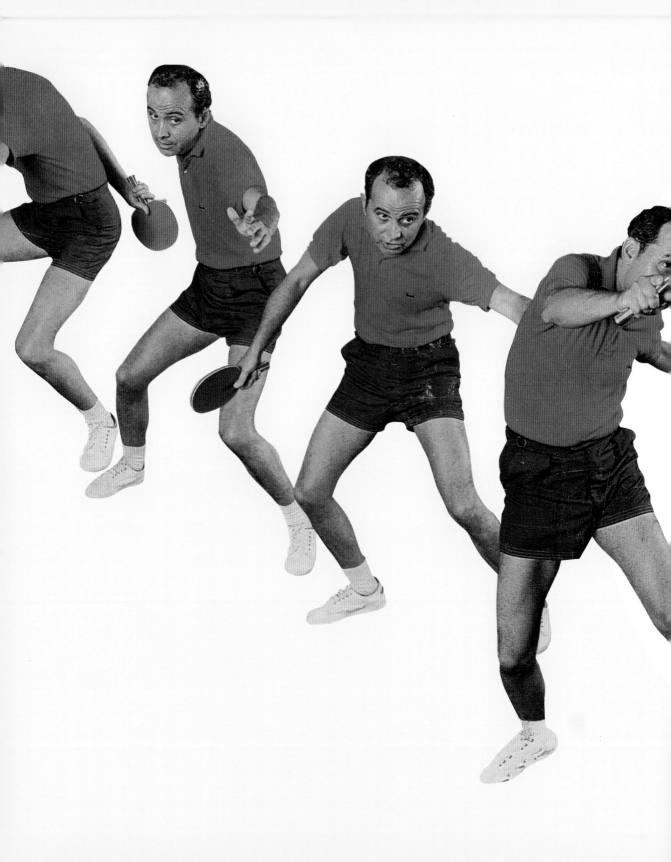

EVERYTHING YOU KNOW IS PONG

HOW MIGHTY TABLE TENNIS SHAPES OUR WORLD

ROGER BENNETT & ELI HOROWITZ

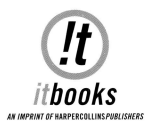

*it*books

AN IMPRINT OF HARPERCOLLINS PUBLISHERS

Inner images: Coleman Clark, Richard Bergmann,
Jill Hammersley, and Dick Miles.

*it***books**

HarperCollins books may be purchased for educational, business, or sales promotional use. For information please write: Special Markets Department, HarperCollins Publishers, 10 East 53rd Street, New York, NY 10022.

FIRST EDITION

Designed by Jayme Yen

Library of Congress Cataloging-in-Publication Data has been applied for.

ISBN 978–0–06–169051–8

10 11 12 13 14 OV/SCPC 10 9 8 7 6 5 4 3 2 1

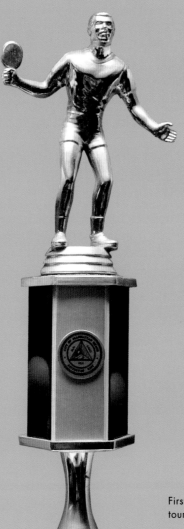

To Nigel and Jamie, with thanks for all the lessons
you taught me on and off the table. And to Eric Kirsch, one of the
greatest the Manchester Jewish Table Tennis League has
ever seen. —RB

To my father and brother, for teaching me how to lose,
and my mother, for tolerating the destruction. —EH

First place trophy for a local ping pong
tournament won by the book designer's father.

CONTENTS

INTRODUCTION X

1

THE LONG GREEN BATTLEFIELD
GEOPOLITICS AND THE SPORT OF KINGS 1
Final Frontiers...22
The Wanderer *by Jesse Aaron Cohen*...............................31

2

IF YOU LIVED HERE,
YOU'D BE RALLYING BY NOW
HOW PING PONG CREATED THE AMERICAN SUBURB.................39
Sun, Sea, and Spin...54
Thoughts from Home *by Jonathan Safran Foer* 61

3

FOREHAND FOREPLAY
AND THE TOPSPIN SEDUCTION
PING PONG AS APHRODISIAC 67
Hits and Ass 84
Tessa *by Davy Rothbart*...93

4

STARS: THEY'RE JUST LIKE US
PING PONG AND CELEBRITY 99
The Library of Champions 112
No Proper Sport *by Nick Hornby*....................................121

THE PADDLE OF YOUTH

5

AGING BODIES, DECAYING MINDS, AND THE QUEST FOR ETERNAL LIFE

AGING BODIES, DECAYING MINDS, AND THE QUEST FOR ETERNAL LIFE.. 125
Health Hazards...140
The Life Pursuit *by Howard Jacobson* 147

THE GREAT BALL OF CHINA

6

PING PONG AND THE CHINESE CENTURY

PING PONG AND THE CHINESE CENTURY 155
Deutschland, Deutschland Über Alles 172
Zen and the Art of Forgetting *by Starlee Kine*....................179

VELOUR COUTURE

7

THE WANING AND WAXING OF PING PONG STYLE

THE WANING AND WAXING OF PING PONG STYLE................ 187
Smash Hits! 204
Out of Fashion *by Harry Evans* 211

AUGMENTED REALITY

8

WHEN PONG BECAME *PONG*, AND EVERYTHING AFTER

WHEN PONG BECAME *PONG*, AND EVERYTHING AFTER 219
A Century of Invention...232
My Quest *by Will Shortz* 243

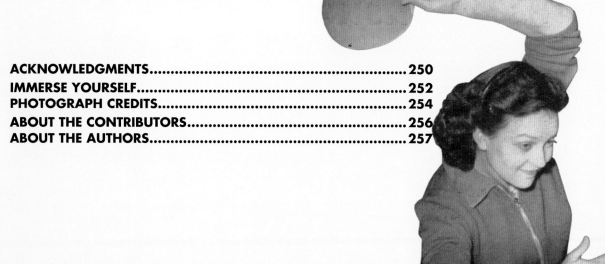

ACKNOWLEDGMENTS..250
IMMERSE YOURSELF..252
PHOTOGRAPH CREDITS..254
ABOUT THE CONTRIBUTORS......................................256
ABOUT THE AUTHORS...257

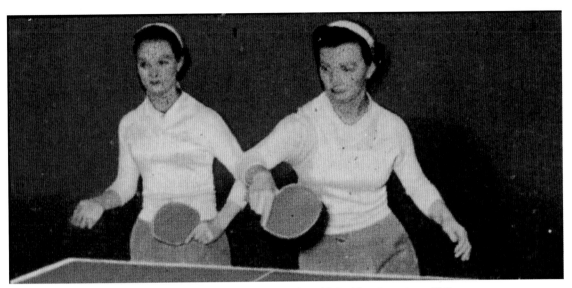

Diane (a lefty) and Rosalind (a righty) Rowe—twins and world doubles champions, 1951.

INTRODUCTION

Every sport claims to be the world's game—soccer, basketball, kabbadi. But few can match the global status acquired by modest yet ubiquitous ping pong: constant but never ascendant, unconcerned with macho posturing, all the while secreting its fingerprints across popular culture. From Fidel Castro to Prince Charles, Thelonious Monk to 50 Cent, George Foreman to Arnold Schwarzenegger, Charlie Chaplin to Ellen DeGeneres—all have clutched a paddle, all have peered across the net with menacing intent. If you throw in a billion hard-core Chinese aficionados, it is no empty boast to claim that ping pong is the most popular yet misunderstood pastime in the world today—the sleeping giant of fast-paced fun.

Ping pong's unvanquished strength lies, paradoxically, in its shabby exterior. Amid the rapid cycles of our world's escalating media omniscience, today's obscure Brazilian hobby becomes tomorrow's Hollywood blockbuster overnight, leaving no time to develop the depth and richness that can be forged only through generations of basement heroics. Neglected by the corporate hunger for the New New New Thing, ping pong has been allowed to flourish in dark corners and distant alleys around the world, nurturing a wealth of lore, legends, and die-hard fans. It is the magma lurking beneath the Earth's crust, piping hot and eternally bubbling.

Other sports may have cross-cultural appeal, but theirs is the appeal of a spreading hegemony; an NBA fan in Shanghai wears the same Melo jersey as an NBA fan in Sheboygan. The power of ping pong, however, lies in its adaptability. Its touch is ubiquitous but gentle—a caress, not a clutch. Neither jihad nor McDonald's, ping pong does not crush local mores nor homogenize for profit, fluttering mothlike to any bright light. It thrives in suburban sheds and Bangkok backrooms, providing a stage upon which countless daily dramas are performed. A global community of a thousand different villages, each a little world in itself—New Jersey rec rooms, Beijing stadia, dwarf child champions, elderly enthusiasts, Hollywood hipsters, perky porn stars—all united by a shared humanity, all noble in their idiosyncrasies. Thomas Freidman claimed that the world is flat; nay, Thomas, we say—the world is round, plastic, and always spinning.

This game brought the two of us together as well: one a chiseler, the other a modified wiper, but joined in a common hunger. When we are not playing the game itself, we can be found immersing ourselves in the ripples left in its wake, amassing a treasury of artifacts unearthed in garages, thrift shops, and archives around the world. From our headquarters on opposite coasts, we have hunted these photos and factoids, the data and detritus, the posters, postcards, and phone cards, driven by a belief that this ever-growing collection offers a glimpse of a hidden kingdom, a realm where culture, politics, love, and war collide. For others, ping pong may amount to little more than a fancy. To us, it is an oracle, a palantir, a Magic 8-Ball that is never wrong.

And so, with the aid of our friends and fellow enthusiasts, it is our honor to present this tale—a story of a thousand smaller stories, a story in which we are all vital characters, a billion tiny balls bouncing back and forth upon an endless globe. Welcome to this world—our world, your world, the world behind the world. A world in which everything you know is pong.

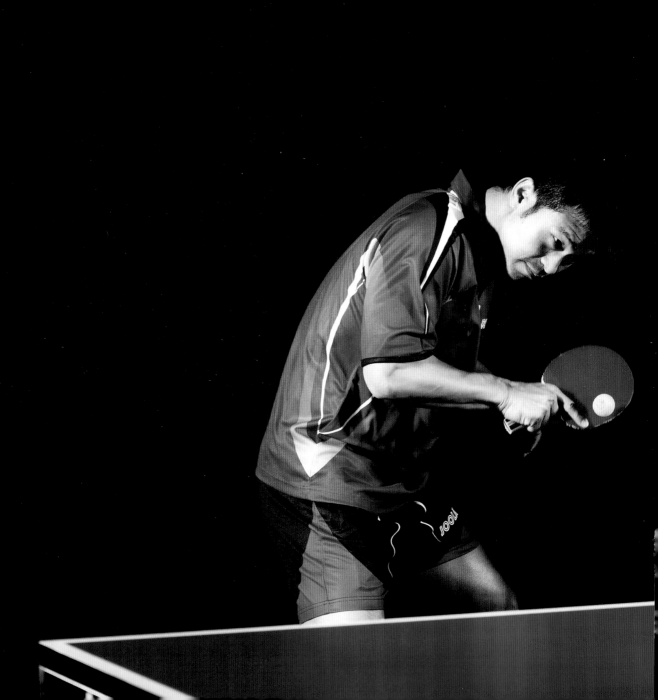

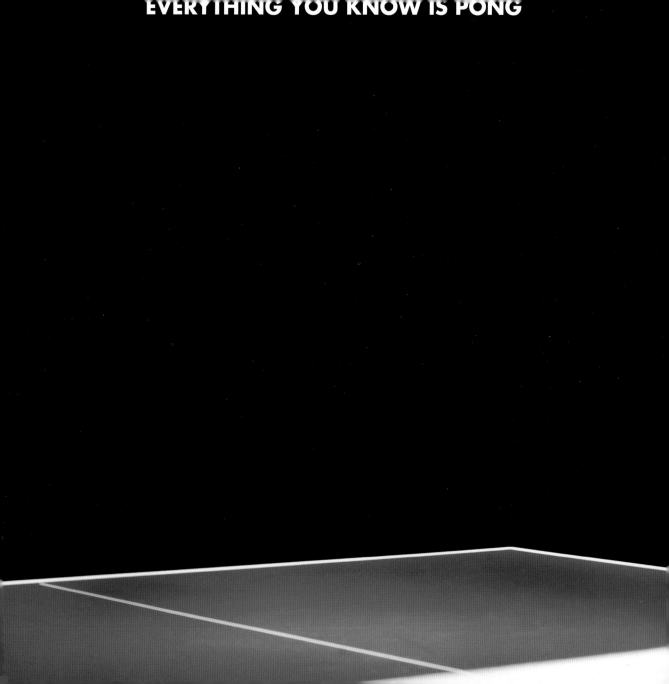
EVERYTHING YOU KNOW IS PONG

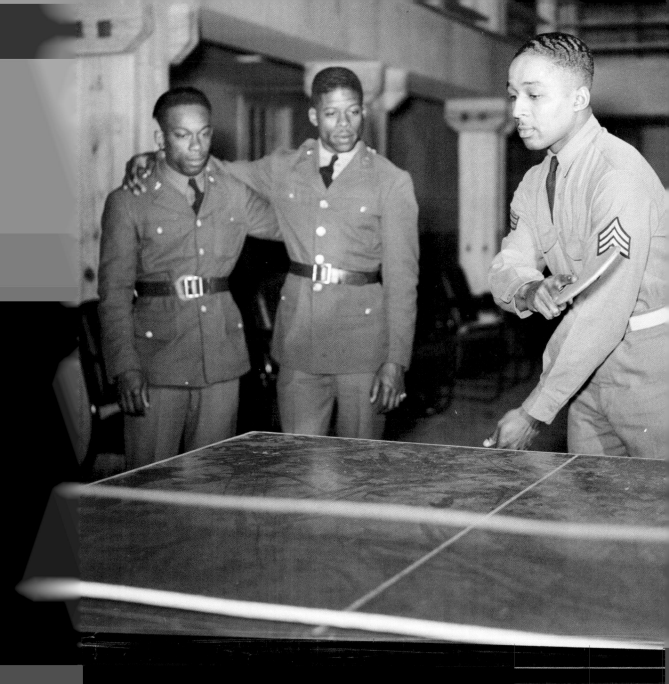

THE LONG GREEN BATTLEFIELD

GEOPOLITICS AND THE SPORT OF KINGS

Ask any junior faculty or armchair historian about ping pong's intersection with the geopolitical trends of the twentieth century, and you're certain to receive a straightened posture, a twitch of bushy eyebrows, and a long ode to Mao, Nixon, Kissinger, and the beloved legend of Ping Pong Diplomacy—the long-overdue thawing of diplomatic relations between the two superpowers, under the safe cover of a harmless sports exchange, innocent athletes in tight shorts providing a lingua sino to transcend cultural barriers. It's a long, colorful story, full of handsome young Americans thrown into a spicy cauldron of international gamesmanship.

Unfortunately, it's also a sham. So-called Ping Pong Diplomacy had very little to do with the game we know and love, and much more to do with those true, perpetual global pastimes: greed and fear. China wanted to cement its

Three soldiers in the service club at Fort Bragg, 1942.

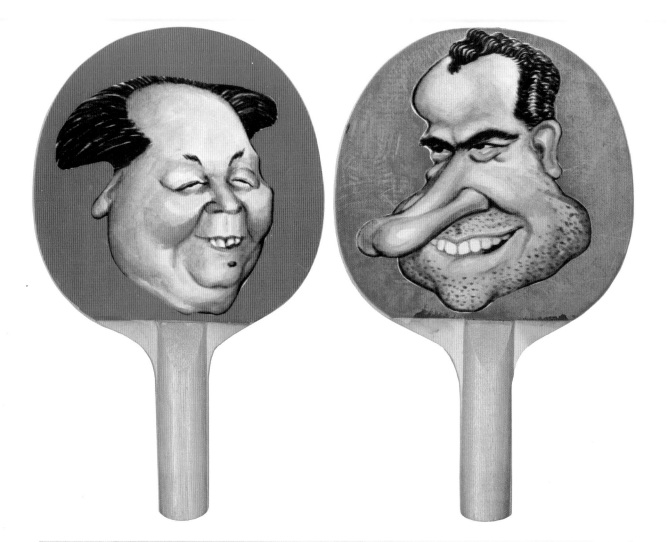

Novelty bats celebrating 1971's Ping Pong Diplomacy.

claim to Taiwan, and the U.S. was terrified of the Soviet foothold in Asia. Ping pong was a wide-eyed innocent just happy for a moment in the spotlight. But this spotlight was in fact a radioactive beam straight to the genitals, for the true effect was not adulation but emasculation; the game we know and love was used as an ignorant sap, a patsy. The athletes were trotted out into brightly lit gymnasiums, but the real action was in the shadows and smoke of the back rooms, the dank lairs of Nixon and Kissinger and their kind. We can imagine them, corpulent and greasy, chuckling in pride at their masterstroke. "Ping pong!" they wheeze. "What could be more harmless than ping pong?" (For an alternate take on this encounter, see page 165.) Little did they know.

The jowly fatcats won the day, but they lost the century; Nixon's corpse began rotting decades before his death, and Kissinger will soon face eternal justice. These men did not know their history, and they have paid the price. The real story of ping pong in the bloody dance of this century gone by cannot be found on a commemorative plate. The truth dwells in darker corners—in Auschwitz, in Guantánamo Bay, in Castro's rebel camps. The field of geopolitics is not a chessboard but a long green table, and the ball never stops bouncing.

We can best understand ping pong as a sort of Forrest Gump of the twentieth century. While Forrest was content to frolic in a playground of babyboomer signifiers—all the way from Woodstock to Washington, wow!—ping pong truly spans the years and the globe. Sometimes buffeted by massive forces, sometimes doing the buffeting itself, two paddles and a ball have been there every step of the way.

The story begins at the end of the previous century, in India, cradle of the purest games of modernity: dice, chess, cockfighting, kabaddi. In this case, however, the invention was not homegrown, but rather a prescient example of cultural fusion. British soldiers, after a long day of colonial exploitation, used cigar-box lids to bat wine corks across tables stacked with books. From these boozy beginnings a behemoth was born. By the turn of the century the fad was spreading across the ballrooms of Europe, Old World aristocrats eagerly co-opting this subcontinental creation. Early names included flim-flam, whiff-whaff, and gossima, until 1901 when Parker Brothers acquired the name Ping-Pong.

Already we've seen early hallmarks of the twentieth century: colonial decay, cultural appropriation, and competing trademarks. Next up was the rise of the immigrant underclass. World War I shattered the gossima delusions of the aristocracy, and the Great Depression humbled the rest. Ping pong provided a cheap, democratic pastime accessible to those who had been excluded from the polo fields of previous centuries. The game proved particularly popular among the Jews of Central Europe; eight of the first nine World Table Tennis Championships were won by Hungary, led by Jewish stars Viktor Barna and Lazlo Bellak. This run was broken in 1936 by Austria, who had found its own Hebrew champ in Richard Bergmann.

But trouble was brewing in Europe, and within three years Bergmann and Barna were teaming up to win the doubles title—for England, their new home. (*The New Yorker* reported that Bergmann "considered Fascism incompatible with the advancement of ping pong and, taking his life in his hands, fled to England, where he is now teaching the game to the British troops.") Those 1939 championships in Cairo were the last until 1947, as the Nazis spread their reign of anti–ping pong hate across Europe. Many of the Jewish stars followed Bergmann and Barna to safer countries, but some were not so lucky—such as Alojzy Ehrlich.

Ehrlich was a Polish Jew and a top player, a three-time runner-up at the World Championships. His legend was secured at the 1936 Swaythling Cup in Prague, when he met Romanian Paneth Farcas in an early round. Both were cautious, defensive players, and it was sure to be a grueling match. Two hours and twelve minutes later, they were finally finished . . . with the first point. During those twelve thousand volleys across the net, the umpire had to be replaced due to a sore neck, Ehrlich began playing left-handed to preserve energy, and an emergency meeting of the International Table Tennis Federation was held—with Ehrlich serving as the Polish representative, mid-rally. Farcas forfeited twenty minutes into the second point, and Ehrlich was on his way to

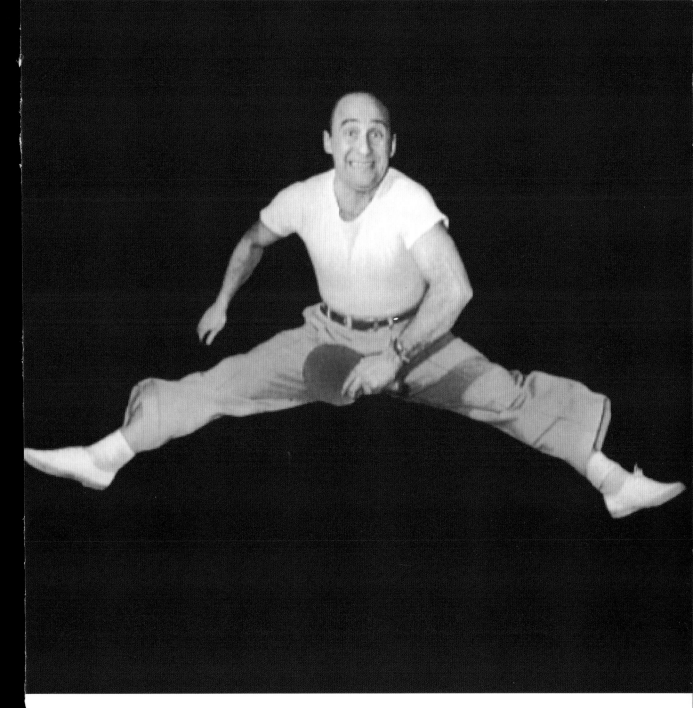

The kings of prewar Europe: Bellak (above), Barna (over, left), and Bergmann (over, right).

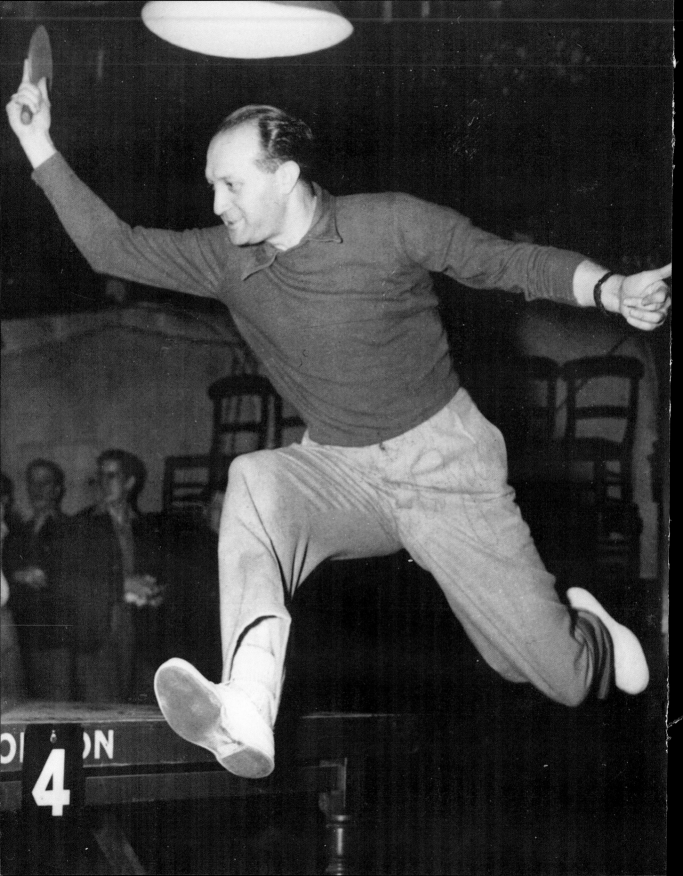

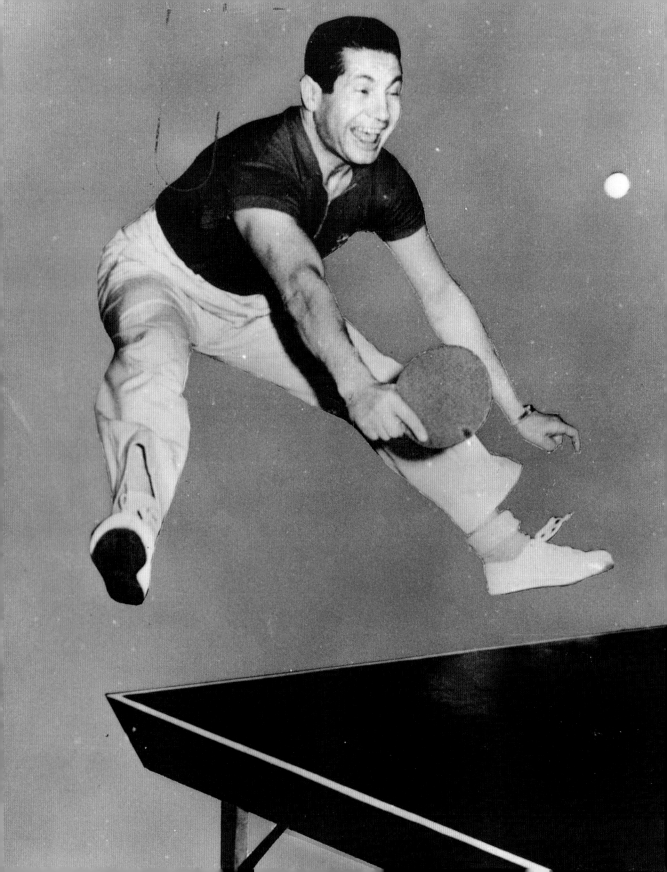

the finals. (For a more in-depth account of this match, please see Dick Miles's riveting article in the November 15, 1965, issue of *Sports Illustrated*.)

This perseverance was tested six years later, when Ehrlich was captured by the Germans and sent to Auschwitz and later Dachau. His six-foot-four frame, ideal for corralling distant slams, now carried only eighty pounds. He was eventually sent to the gas chamber—but then was spared when a guard recognized him from tournament heroics. Ehrlich managed to outlast the war and even returned to the World Championships in 1957, now representing France.

Meanwhile, back in the U.S. of A., ping pong was experiencing sunnier times as a central part of the American war effort. In previous decades, the military had taken a firm antipong stance, a product of benighted notions of traditional masculinity evidenced by Major General John F. O'Ryan, commander of the National Guard. In 1914, O'Ryan embarked upon a campaign to toughen the Guard, declaring, "Ballroom soldiers and ping pong warriors are not wanted in the National Guard. If we advertised for ping pong soldiers

New York Times, January 12, 1915, page 5.

GOVERNOR HEARS PROTESTS OF 22D

But Intimates That O'Ryan's Reorganization Order Will Be Carried Out.

PING-PONG CHARGE HURTS

Heated Speeches Delyivered Against That and "Dance-Hall" Epithet —Name to be Preserved.

Special to The New York Times.

ALBANY, Jan. 11.—Gov. Whitman tonight told a delegation representing the Twenty-second Regiment of Engineers of New York thta the name and headquarters of the regiment would be preserved but intimated that the

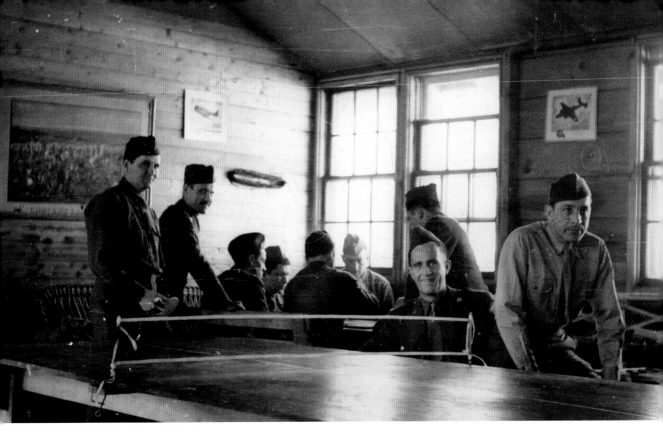

"Ping pong warriors" paused in a rare moment of rest: American soldiers during World War II.

and offered them dances as an inducement to join, we could get more men than we wanted. We want in the National Guard strong, athletic, and intelligent men who enjoy camping and roughing it."

Reaction was swift and angry. Many veterans spoke up in favor of dancing, one arguing that "on the night before the battle of Waterloo the Allies had a dance. Napoleon was overthrown the next day"; another, eighty-five-year-old Colonel John B. Silliman, said, "I dance myself when I get a chance, and it doesn't hurt a good soldier. The more ladies around the armory, the more men." Unfortunately, while many defended dancing, they objected only to the *accusations* of ping pong; in those early misguided years, the sport was seen as footloose frippery. A *New York Times* headline proclaimed "Ping-Pong Charge Hurts," and soldiers scurried to prove their antipong credentials. (Don't Ask, Don't Tell seems almost *enlightened* in comparison.)

That was late 1914, as the United States closed its eyes and ears to the mounting turmoil in Europe. By 1919, however, the War to End All Wars was a fact of life, and all pretenses were stripped away; macho pongaphobia was a luxury our military could no longer afford. The *Times* now reported: "Ping pong is coming to be the favorite sport of the American Expeditionary Force over there." Six weeks later the Treaty of Versailles was signed. Ping pong warriors had won in the end.

Thus, by the time World War II rolled in, ping pong was firmly established as a wholesome, manly endeavor, a favored pastime on army bases, and a reassuring reminder of normalcy while awaiting deployment to foreign shores. Ping pong was also contributing to the war effort behind closed doors. A top secret military installation known only as P.O. Box 1142 (its mailing address in northern Virginia) interrogated almost 4,000 German prisoners of war, using a variety of enlightened—and effective—techniques. In a quote that sent ripples through the modern table-tennis military-intelligence community, ninety-one-year-old Henry Kolm, a veteran of the World War II intelligence efforts, recently said, "We got more information out of a German general with a game of chess or ping pong than they do today, with their torture."

Of course, not all cultural exchange was so well intentioned. Any weapon as powerful as a smiling pongeur runs the risk of abuse; any potent symbol can be deployed as a false signifier. And such was the case on our own shores, in the Japanese internment camps. In our government's queasy, ambivalent reasoning, the Japanese-Americans were possible spies, but also friends and neighbors; they couldn't just *run free*, but they shouldn't *suffer*. How to communicate to the nation that these "war relocation camps" weren't anything to worry about? The easy solution: elaborately staged proponganda photos. See, folks? It's a *camp*—fun!

The war ends. Peace, sort of, reigns. And here enters one of the most controversial, committed pongeurs of the twentieth century: Fidel Castro. In 1951 Castro was just a young lawyer running for the legislature, attempting to contribute to a new Cuba. Early in 1952, however, two events reshaped Castro's political philosophy and forged his revolutionary destiny. The second

"Manzanar, California: These girls are enjoying a game of ping pong in a girls' recreation center at this War Relocation Authority center for evacuees of Japanese ancestry."

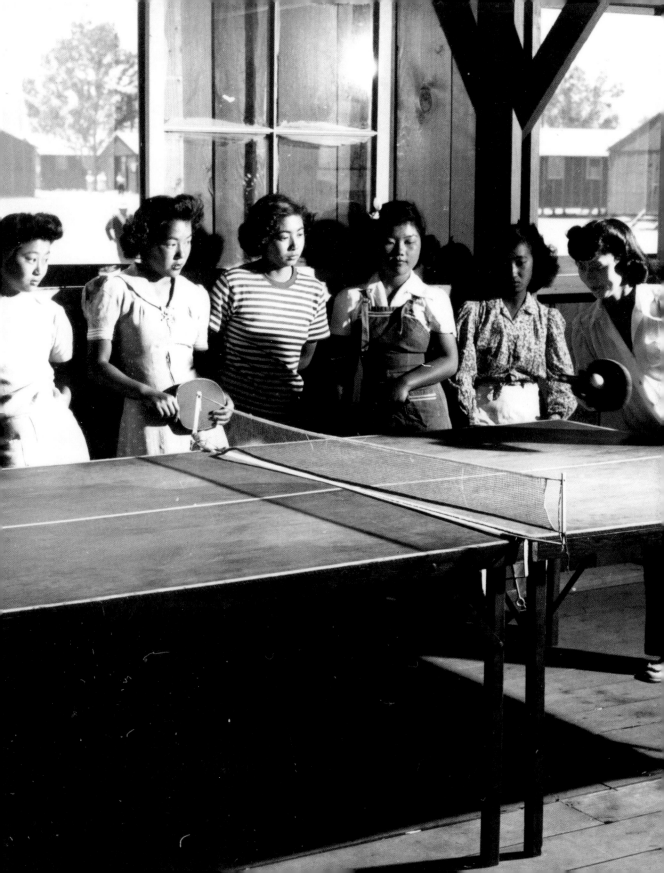

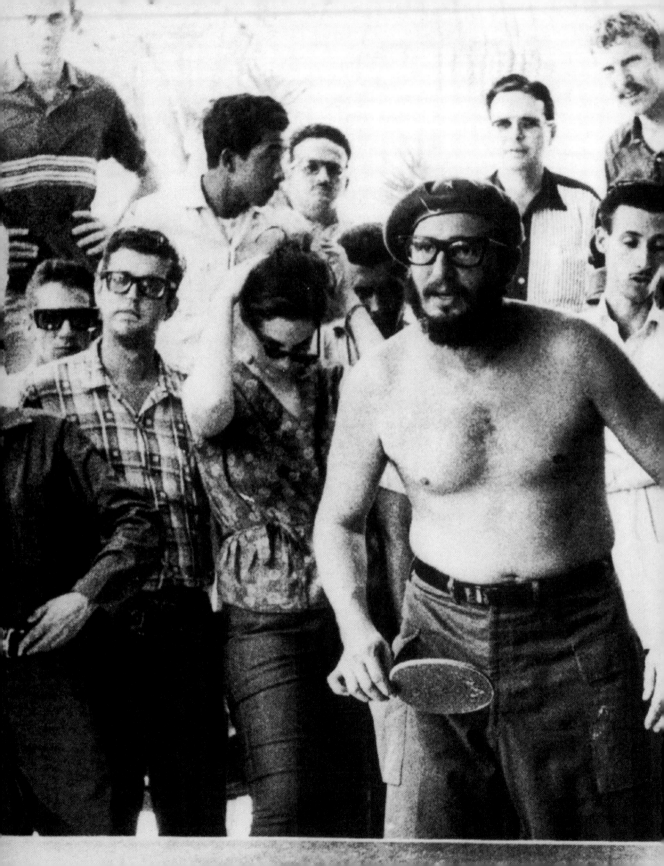

event is widely known: Batista's military coup on March 10, which eliminated Castro's hopes of changing the government from the inside. Just a month before, however, came an uprising of a different sort, one that sent shock waves through ping pong circles worldwide and showed Fidel how innovation and insouciance can be used to upend even the most dominant opponent. I refer, of course, to Hiroji Satoh's debut of the sponge-bat at the 1952 World Championships in Bombay. Satoh was an unheralded player, scrawny and nearsighted, not even top-three on his own Japanese team. But in Bombay he unveiled a thick, soft paddle, capable of absorbing even the slammiest slam and intensifying his opponent's own spin—in effect, using the enemy's power against him. Satoh went on to win the world title that February, upsetting the razor-sharp, needle-thin Marty Reisman in a historic match that haunts the American table-tennis community to this day. According to traditionalists, the sponge-bat ruined ping pong forever—but to Fidel Castro, it must have been a revelation, and perhaps an inspiration. Three months later Castro fled to the mountains and began planning his revolution.

The following year he launched his first attack, on the Moncada Barracks, but it failed miserably; Castro had absorbed Satoh's revolutionary spirit but still was at a loss for specific *tactics*. Castro was imprisoned and then was exiled in early 1955. By 1957, however, he was back in Cuba, having relaunched the ultimately successful revolution we know and love today. What happened during that exile to transform Castro's struggling strategy? The answer lies in midtown Manhattan.

In November of 1955 Castro traveled to New York to raise funds for his movement. He delivered a rousing speech before a crowd of 800 at the Palm Garden Hall, 306 West Fifty-second Street, and the dollars rolled in. This much is known. What is not known, but is much speculated upon, is what he did next—*immediately* next. Castro's schedule for the day is lost to history, but does it not seem likely that he might have fled the gilded ballroom for more familiar surroundings? Imagine young Fidel, twenty-nine years old, stepping out on the streets of New York City. He heads one block east. Turns left on Broadway. Does Fidel wrinkle his nose at the rampant capitalism? No

Castro on the battlefield, Havana, 1963.

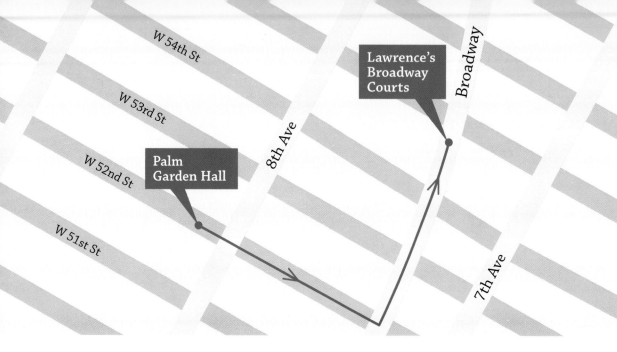

Fidel Castro's hypothesized pilgrimage, 1955.

matter—this night is no longer about politics. He heads north, one block, two
. . . and then sees the holy ground he has been seeking: Lawrence's Broadway
Courts, a table tennis emporium in an old Legs Diamond speakeasy (previously known as the Nutty Club). Lawrence's was the sweaty center of American
ping pong, the legendary battleground of Dick Miles, Lou Pagliaro, and Marty
Reisman himself, still smarting from his loss to Satoh three years before. Here
the play was furious, passionate, and utterly individual. And perhaps Reisman's
quintessentially New York game—a crafty, razor-sharp blend of spin, speed,
precision, and chatter—taught Fidel what Satoh's victory could not.

Castro left the United States, rejoined Che and the guerillas, and declared
his new strategy: "Like ping pong," he said, "you hit them where they least
expect it." (This is what he said!) They headed for the Sierra Maestra mountains and began a Reisman-like campaign of unexpected strikes from the
depths of the jungle. Three years later, Castro's army was celebrating in the
streets of Havana.

Castro never forgot the source of his victory. Twelve years into his regime,
with the aforementioned sham of Ping Pong Diplomacy gobbling up the

airwaves, he was asked, "Would you accept a ping pong game Nixon?" Fidel's reply: "I have better competitors with whom to play ping pong." This was a man who understood that the long green battlefield was not to be trifled with.

The midcentury arrival of Satoh's sponge-bat signaled changes beyond the Cuban Revolution. We can see its echoes in the ensuing Cold War arms race, the equipment becoming more important than the soldier/player. There are also early glimmers of the Eastward power shift to come in the following decades. Japan and China were emerging from the ashes of war, and Satoh's shocking upset foreshadowed the imminent Asian dominance of consumer electronics and small paddle/racket sports (with occasional competition from northern Europe in both areas). Meanwhile the U.S. descended into uncertain wars and intergenerational bickering, and our tables descended into our bomb

A bomb shelter promotional postcard, circa 1960, capturing the emasculated state of post-heyday, pre-rebirth North American table tennis.

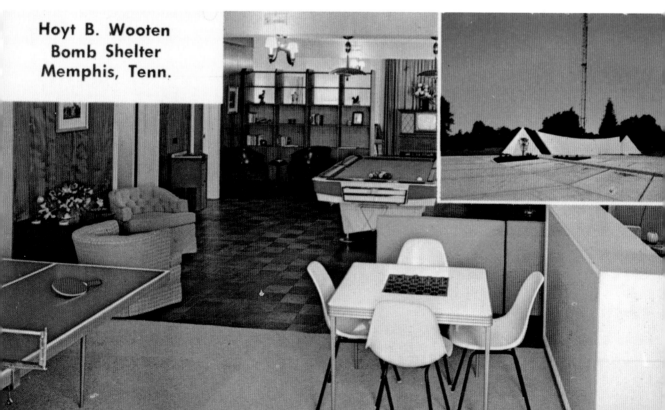

Hoyt B. Wooten
Bomb Shelter
Memphis, Tenn.

shelters. The next fifty years were lost to consumerism and fear. And so the twentieth century came to close—in with a ping, out with a whimper.

The game's specter, however, stretches farther than ever. Francis Fukuyama famously proclaimed "the end of history," but the pong goes on. We see its presence in Saudi "jihad rehab" centers, which use table tennis to draw young militants away from Al Qaeda. We see its absence in Abu Ghraib, where the enlightened interrogation tactics of World War II have been replaced by crude, pongless torture and humiliation. We see its persistent power as a symbol of pure freedom in the case of Ratko Mladic, an accused Serbian war criminal on the lam; Mladic had been observed dancing, delivering wedding toasts, and getting into a snowball fight, but the appearance that enraged the international community is when he was witnessed playing ping pong in an army barracks. (Repercussions were swift and wide; the *UN Dispatch* asked: "Could Ratko Mladic playing ping pong hurt Serbia's EU chances?") Modern asymmetric warfare seems to have taken Castro's advice one step further, mirroring ping pong's contrarian, persistent survival: decentralized cells, makeshift facilities, and unpredictable techniques, a rebuke to technocrats and capitalists.

A paddle is only as good as the player who wields it. What this world needs now is a leader who can bind the power of pong to the forces of freedom. Many have tried; the movers and shakers of the twentieth century traded in their polo mallets for rubber paddles, echoing the populist era. The results have not always been pretty, but they are inevitably revealing. Castro, we have discussed, and Chairman Mao is obvious, but the pong pantheon includes telling portraits of Vladimir Putin, all steely determination and tight buttocks; Lech Walesa, full of humane zeal; and Yasser Arafat and his men, torn between the paddle and the pistol; Tony Blair and Prince Charles, displaying their respective slippery opportunism and limp-wristed gentility; and our beloved Clintons, bursting with baby boomer overenthusiasm. Nicholas Sarkozy of France, Richard Lagos of Chile, Kwame Nkrumah of Ghana, Goren

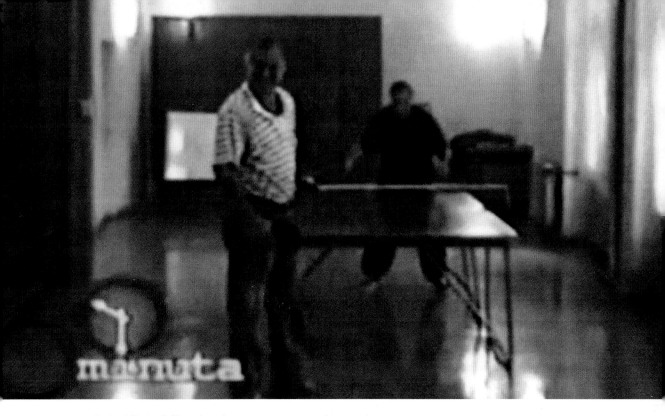

Ratko Mladic (left) in the infamous, incriminating home video.

Persson of Sweden, Denis Sassou-Nguesso of Congo, Luis Inacio Lulu da Silva of Brazil—all have awkwardly approached a table for that invaluable photo op. Why waste time shaking hands or kissing babies? A few chipper volleys provide all the same benefits, without the collateral dangers of assassination or swine flu.

But now the paddle has been passed to a new generation. What of our current Hopemonger-in-Chief? Daughters Sasha and Malia recently defeated Nick Jonas backstage at the *Ellen DeGeneres Show*, but there are no known photos of Obama himself with a paddle in hand. His commitment to the cause is well established, however; as an Illinois state senator, he directed government funds to support the 2004 U.S. Open in Chicago, and then addressed a congratulatory letter to his "dear table tennis friends." Bizarrely, Obama's critics attempt to use this behind-the-scenes ping pong advocacy *against* him. *The Case Against Barack Obama* declares: "Perhaps the most surprising story

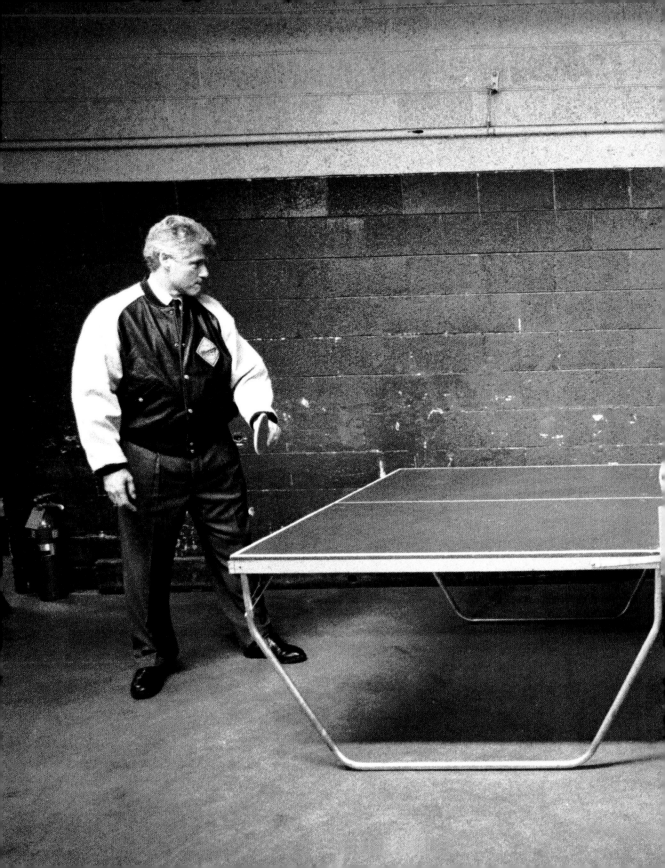

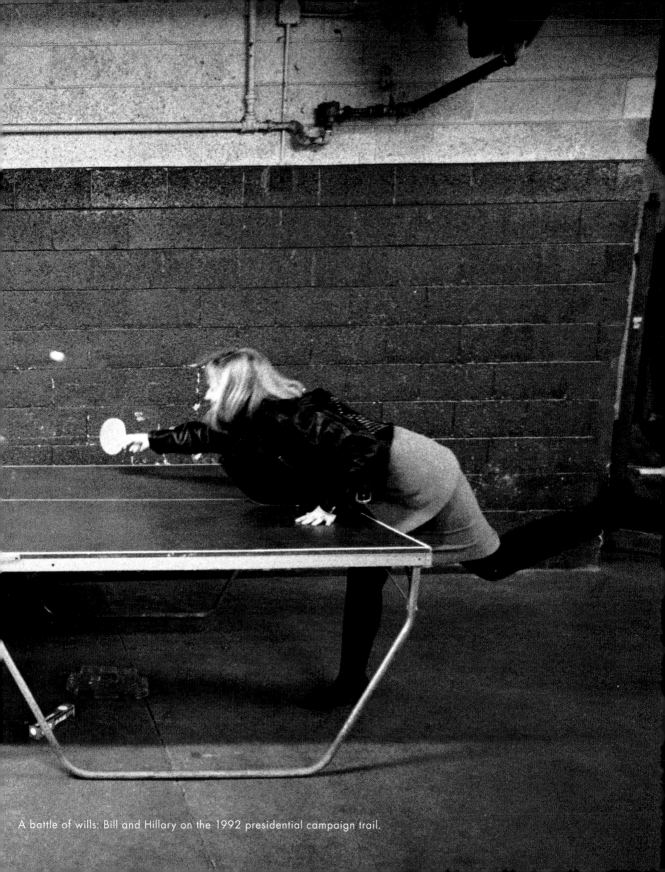

A battle of wills: Bill and Hillary on the 1992 presidential campaign trail.

about Barack Obama and money is the one that no one talks about at all. It involves ping pong." We agree: people *should* talk about this. After so much struggle, after a century of bloodshed and hostility, it is time for the truth to be heard. It is time to come out of the basements and rec rooms and bomb shelters, time to step out into the sunshine. Perhaps Barack Obama can be the one to finally cleanse our nation's sins, shattering that historical barrier: our first true Ping Pong President. A new day dawns.

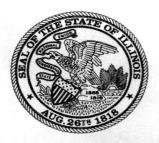

Illinois State Senator Barack Obama

1013 East 53rd Street
Chicago, Illinois 60615
(773) 363-1996

June 30, 2004

Dear Table Tennis Friends:

This letter is to express my enthusiasm for the SPINvitational and the Killerspin U.S. Open in Chicago during the week of June 30 through July 3. The City of Chicago plans to partner with the State of Illinois to make this an extremely successful international event that will help promote business and tourism in Chicago.

The SPINvitational will be broadcast on ESPN television in 156 countries and viewed by tens of millions of people and it continues your efforts to make Chicago the table tennis capital of this nation. The State of Illinois and the City of Chicago will be supporting the SPINvitational with several major promotional efforts.

Table tennis remains one of the top sports in the world and the activity continues to pick up steam. Table tennis is a major U.S. sport with 2.2 million frequent participants and 20 million total participants. Worldwide, more than 300 million people play table tennis. Table tennis is the top rated sport for TV viewership in China and China is one of the world's only growing financial and economic markets.

Good luck to all the participants and I want to thank Governor Blagojevich, Department of Commerce and Economic Opportunity Director Jack Lavin, Mayor Daley and everyone else who organized this fine event.

Sincerely,

Barack Obama
State Senator, 13th District

Final Frontiers

Ping pong is, of course, popular not only among presidents, kings, and revolutionaries; it is fundamentally a game of the people. In fact, it may be this ubiquity and demographic-defying appeal that have drawn vote-hungry politicians to the sport. But these ping pong populists can't take the game away from us. Like life itself, ping pong finds its way into every unlikely corner, anywhere, anyone, anything: priests and whores, bunnies and birds, chiefs and bushmen, naked and clothed, with bricks and palms, on mountaintops and in shark-infested waters.

Within the incredible diversity of ping pong ethnopictology, there are two central, opposing strains: hegemony and globalism. In the first, we are presented with a pair of exotic characters in foreign garb, clutching paddles like suburban teens; the goal is to underscore the reach of our culture (with ping pong as its purest symbol), manifest destiny extending to the darkest lands. In the second, the message is one of diversity and communion—peoples of all colors and shapes, united in a shared joy, charmingly resourceful in our local variations (bricks for nets, hands for paddles, etc).

The final image in this collection, however, points toward a third, transcendent strain: intergalactic exchange. Perhaps this could signal ping pong's true role in mankind's future—neither a tentacle of Western culture nor a widespread frivolity, but a bold exploration, a smash toward the stars.

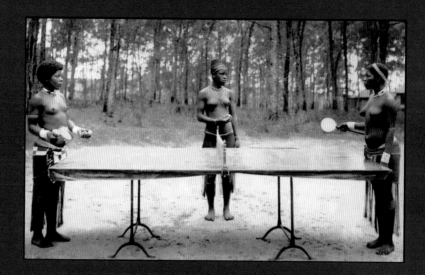

An early example of ping pong imperialism: "Zulu Maidens."

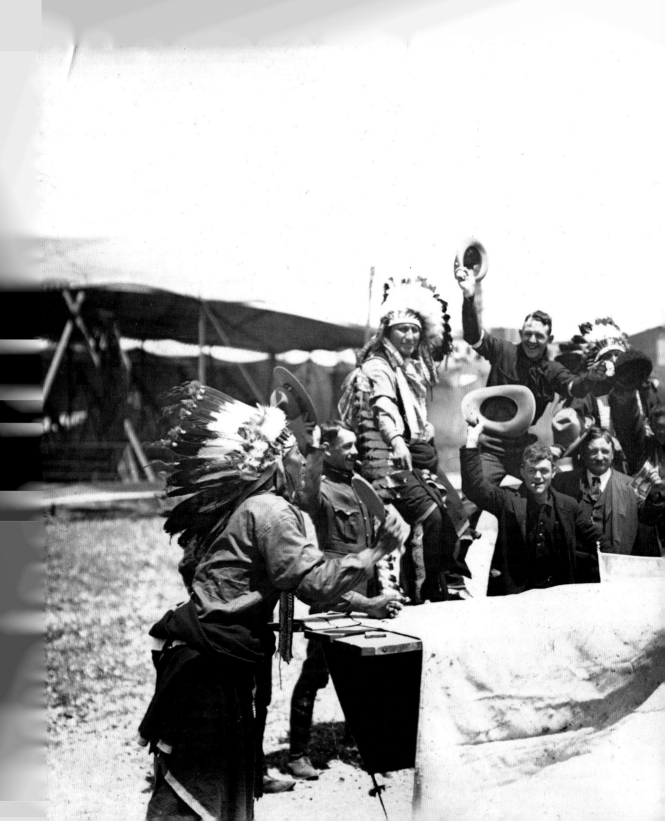

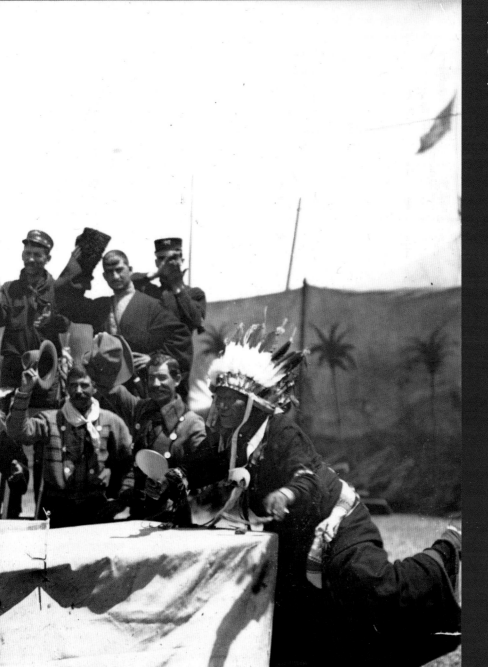

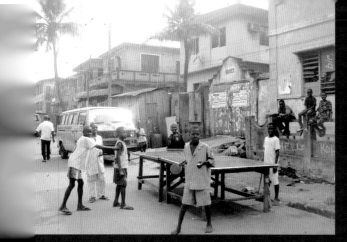

Top: Curbside action in Lagos, Nigeria.
Bottom: Rural Chinese youth: one paddle, no net, no problem.

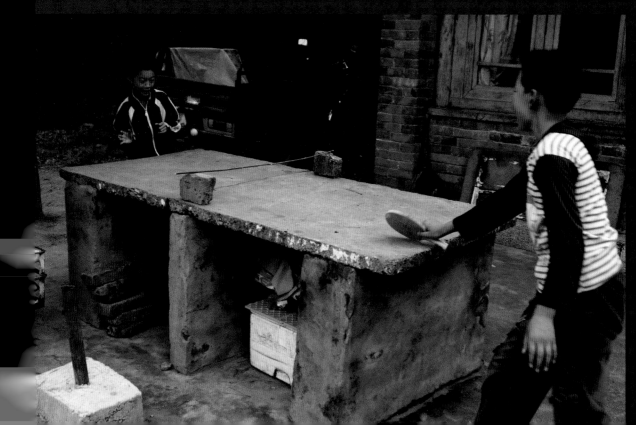

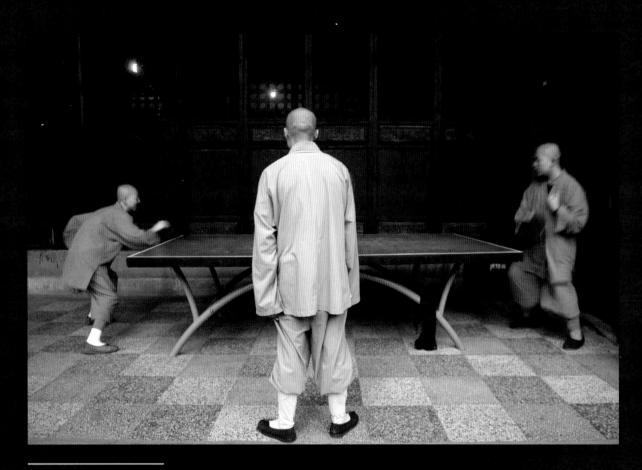

Buddhist monks at a
monastery in Chengdu,
China.

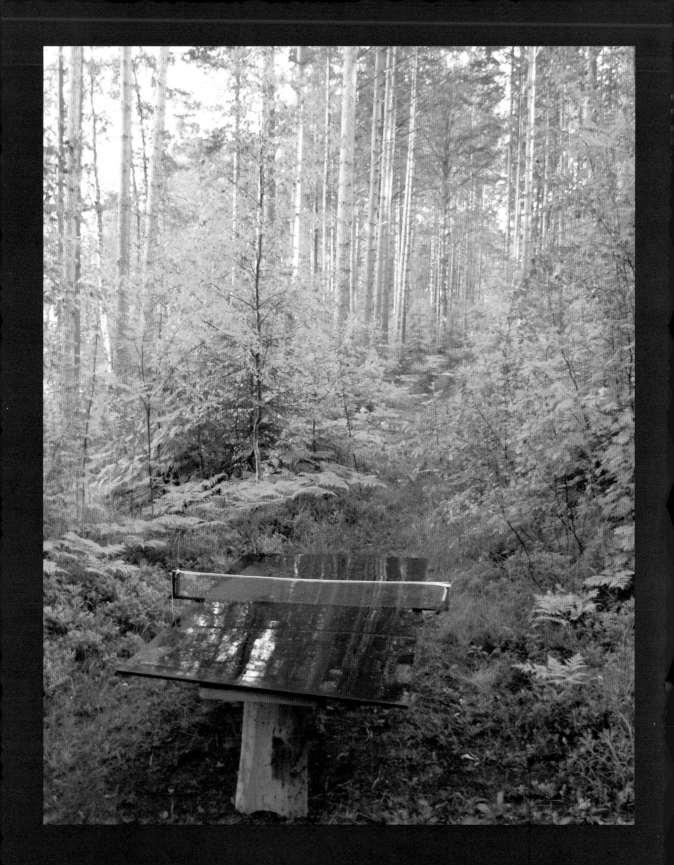

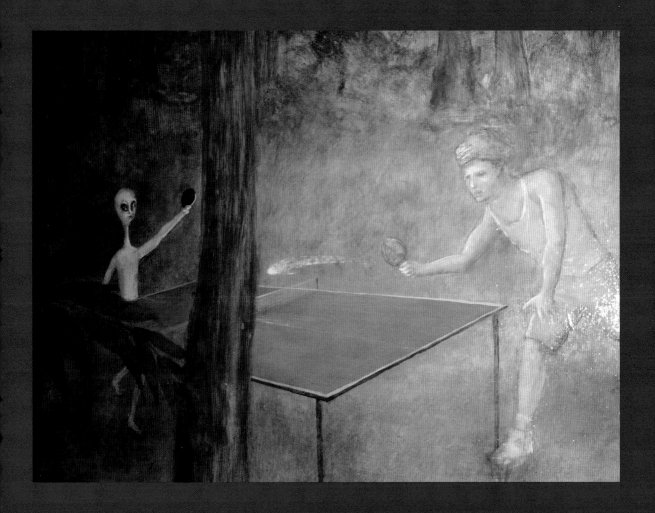

Top: A prescient mural at Comet Ping Pong pizzeria in Washington, D.C.

Left: An oasis in central Finland.

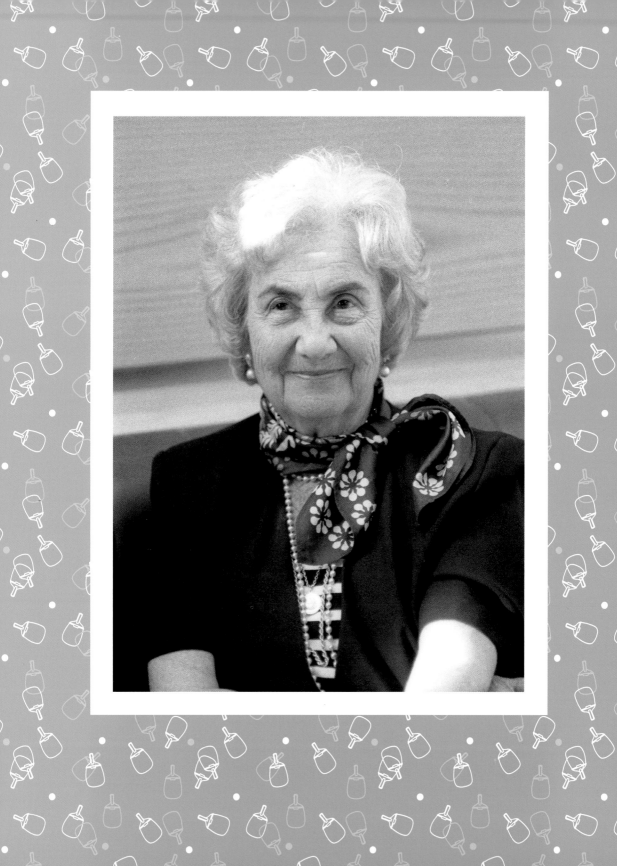

THE WANDERER
BY JESSE AARON COHEN

When I was twenty-four years old, I took a job as a research assistant at a Yiddish library and archives in Manhattan, spending my days in 1920s Warsaw and my nights in 2000s New York. I never set out to become conversant in this fairly obscure history, but I found I enjoyed spending my days reading about the countless, often moving, stories of ordinary people in extraordinary circumstances, all but forgotten now, their letters and correspondence sitting in untouched boxes on the eleventh story of a windowless building on Sixteenth Street. There was the Orthodox Jewish jurist who served in Lenin's first government and then went on to try to persuade the government of Suriname to set up a non-Zionist Jewish state there. There was the American immigrant who edited a Yiddish newspaper, wrote several plays, translated Tolstoy, sued Henry Ford, and served as the American ambassador to Albania in the early 1930s. There was the Ukrainian Jewish watchmaker who was acquitted by a French jury after confessing to the assassination of the national leader of the Ukraine in a sensational 1920s trial.

But the story that stayed with me the most was the saga of Angelica Rozeanu, the Romanian table tennis star who is now widely considered to be the greatest female player of all time. I grew up playing table tennis with my father every night after dinner in the suburban basement of the home where I was raised. Losing night after night was something of a rite of passage. Among my friends, where competition was fierce, ping pong skills were the most highly prized in a triumvirate of activities that also included video baseball and Spit. I think it appealed to me mostly because it was the only sport in which I was not totally afraid of the ball, but I quickly grew tired of losing every night and developed an adolescent personality that shunned competitive sports. I moved on to worrying about bands, girls, and politics.

Angelica Rozeanu, who came of age in a Europe on the brink of catastrophe, also encountered table tennis at a young age, but then she clung to it, mastered it, and eventually held on to it for dear life as she used those skills to survive everything that life could possibly throw at a person. Her extraordinary story is that of a woman and her unparalleled talent amid the violence and upheaval of twentieth-century history. It's an Eastern European *Forrest Gump* in which the theme of the infallibility of virtue is replaced with absurdity, authoritarian regimes, and unending loss. Maybe it's a combination of *Forrest Gump* and Anne Frank.

I first encountered Rozeanu's name while aimlessly flipping through a Mylar-jacketed copy of the *Encyclopedia of Jews in Sports* in the archives' library. It is one of only a few, mostly sadly titled, reference books to include an entry on Rozeanu, whose story has been largely undocumented. In fact, the only source that I was able to track down in which Rozeanu tells her own story is a heartbreaking letter mailed to former U.S. champion Marty Reisman, later printed in the Fall 2001 issue of *Classic HardBat News*, an electronic newsletter for a niche group of classic table tennis enthusiasts.

Angelica Adelstein was born in 1921 to a bourgeois, assimilated Jewish family in Bucharest. When she was eight years old, she came down with a case of scarlet fever; while convalescing at home, her brother Gaston, seven years her senior, returned one day with table tennis balls, paddles, and a net. He proceeded to teach her the basics of the game on their dining room table. Two years later, when a YMCA opened across the street, Angelica began playing and practicing with much stronger players, honing her skills and sharpening her emerging talent. By age fifteen, she won the Romanian National Women's Championship, a title she held continuously until 1957, with the exception of the war years.

Her star rose rapidly. In 1938 she won the Hungarian Open, her first major international victory. She had hoped to travel to London in the same year for the World Championships but was denied a visa by an increasingly right-leaning and openly anti-Semitic Romanian government.

In 1939 she was allowed to travel to Cairo for the Worlds, where she was eliminated by the reigning world champion Vlasta Depetrisova ("in five sets, losing the final game 22–20, with a net-dribbler"). Shortly after her return to Bucharest, conditions at home spiraled downward as Romania allied itself with Nazi Germany. A law was passed banning Jews from athletic centers. "Where are you going to play now, Angelica?" Rozeanu recalled people mockingly asking her in the streets. When the war reached Romania, and the massacres, deportations, and bombardments began, Rozeanu and her family spent four years in hiding, selling their possessions and knitting cheap clothes to support themselves. She played no table tennis.

Following the war, Angelica married Louis "Lulu" Rozeanu and soon gave birth to a daughter. She slowly began to approach the game again, training against strong opponents. In 1948, after a ten-year absence during what should have been the prime of her career, she finally emerged on the international stage at the World Championships at Wembley, where she lost a nail-biter to reigning champion Gizella Farkas.

Life in postwar, Soviet-controlled Romania was difficult for the Rozeanus, and later that year they made an unsuccessful attempt to defect. Arrested and detained near the Hungarian border, they were eventually released and returned to Bucharest, with no money and their reputations tarnished. Angelica was denied a visa to attend the 1949 World Championships, instead eking out a living in Bucharest as a sportswriter for a local newspaper.

With the following year's World Championships held in Hungary, she was allowed to return to international competition, where her fortunes began to rise. Prior to the war, Rozeanu had employed a graceful, defensive style, but the intervening decade had changed her somehow. Perhaps conscious of all the years that had passed her by, Rozeanu came to Budapest with an aggressive, attacking approach, and this vaulted her to the top. The title was her first of a still-unmatched six consecutive singles championships.

Returning to Bucharest a champion, Angelica was showered with titles, awards, and gifts. She was named president of the Romanian Table Tennis Commission; two years later, after winning her third straight singles title in Bombay, she was named head coach of the Romanian national team. In 1953 she made her first of three tours to the Soviet Union, working to popularize the sport there. The government even gave her a car, a rare distinction at the time.

Even through this extraordinary run, which included an unprecedented seventeen world titles in all, ominous signs loomed. She lived under the strict surveillance of the distrustful Communist authorities and its secret police, with agents trailing her at all international events. She was instructed not to talk to any other athletes, lest she be banned from participating in future events.

Seeking her seventh straight singles title at the 1956 Worlds in Tokyo, Angelica met an unknown thirty-two-year-old housewife named Kiyoko Tasaka in a match that some consider to be the greatest in the history of table tennis. After Tasaka took the first two games by scores of 21–19 and 22–20, the other players and umpires throughout the arena joined the 12,000 spectators at Tokyo Coliseum to watch as the final game stretched on and on. When the score reached 30, an ill-equipped scoreboard was rendered unusable.

Tasaka eventually prevailed 32–30. Rozeanu called the defeat the most devastating of her career.

The defeat foreshadowed an end to this period of relative stability, and soon the repressive forces of the paranoid state reemerged. In 1958 the chairmanship of the Romanian National Table Tennis Federation was given to a Party member who quickly enacted a purge of Jewish table tennis players. Rozeanu was accused of engaging in "the cult of personality" and was stripped of her coaching position and forbidden from participating in international competitions.

This treatment continued until 1960, when the chairman himself was purged. While attending a Woman's Day function at the opera, Angelica had a Gumpian chance encounter with Gheorghe Gheorghiu-Dej, then general secretary of the Romanian Communist Party. Angelica, who had been denied access to any important officials, explained to him all that she had endured, confiding that she believed her treatment had something to do with her husband's attempt to leave the country ten years earlier. Gheorghiu-Dej was astonished by the story and instructed her to divorce her husband at once; he would be allowed to leave the country, and she could return to political favor.

Taking the general secretary's advice, Angelica divorced her husband, who then immigrated to Israel, and returned to international competition. Desperate and weary from the horrible highs and lows of life under the fickle and violent regime, she traveled to Vienna to visit her friend, rival, and sometimes doubles partner Trude Pritzi—and never returned. Instead, Angelica and her daughter defected to Israel, leaving behind all of her possessions, medals, and trophies. When her escape was discovered, the Romanian authorities promptly recalled all of the honors and titles that had been bestowed on her.

Reunited with her husband, Angelica settled near Haifa and began a new life without friends, money, or knowledge of the language. She also found herself plopped down in the middle of a new and still-asserting-itself Israeli society, one that was concerned more with the task of creating a new national culture than with preserving the heterogeneity of its populace. Though Angelica easily won the title in table tennis at the 1961 Maccabiah games, Israel's top competition, she was unhappy playing in her new home, feeling that the other players were against her for being "too European." When she was told by Israeli sporting officials in 1962 that it would be too expensive to send her abroad to compete, Angelica, angry and disappointed, gave up playing the sport forever. It would be the last, and most bitterly ironic, government-imposed injustice of her career. In 1969 she took a position at the Elbit computer manufacturing facility in Haifa, which she held through retirement in the early 1980s.

In her retirement years, she told Reisman, "I have scheduled my life so I am busy all the time, so as not to think of what happened in the past, because it doesn't make me feel well. I hope that after I write to you all of this, it won't bring too much of it back to me."

She died in 2006, at the age of eighty-four.

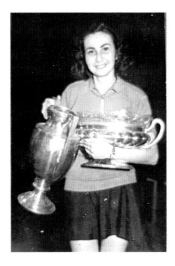

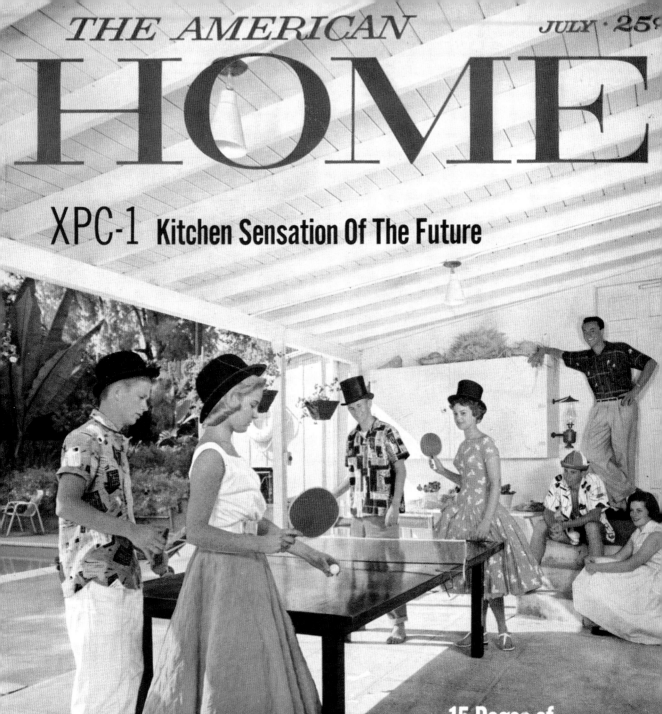

THE AMERICAN
HOME

JULY · 25¢

XPC-1 Kitchen Sensation Of The Future

**15 Pages of
Delicious Hot Weather Food**

GORGEOUS 9 x 12 BIRD PRINT

IF YOU LIVED HERE, YOU'D BE RALLYING BY NOW

HOW PING PONG CREATED THE AMERICAN SUBURB

In the 1950s the United States added one more achievement to those self-declared in "The Star-Spangled Banner." Not content with being just the land of the free and the home of the brave, America took a bold leap toward homogeneity and front lawns, becoming the world's first suburban nation. In the postwar period, the demobilization of sixteen million GIs conspired with the widespread availability of land, the low cost of construction, and the rapid evolution of transport technology to ensure that ownership of a single-family home, previously the status equivalent of a Black Amex card, was available to all. A mortgage became the most potent symbol of unlimited prosperity.

Domestic bliss on the cover of *American Home* magazine, July 1957.

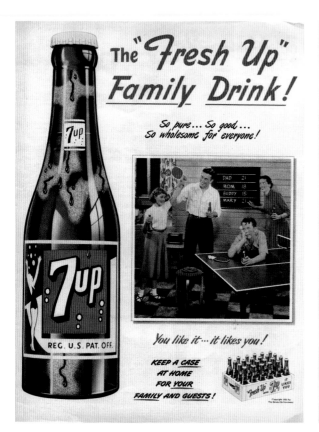

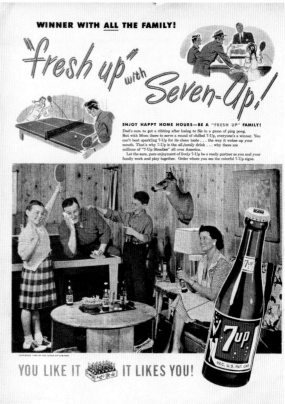

Dad is destroyed as Mom keeps score in these 7Up advertisements from the 1950s.

American cities were quickly turned inside out. In world centers from Paris to Rome, Rio to Bombay, ritzy neighborhoods had traditionally been located in the center, with the slums scattered toward the periphery. This rule of thumb was inverted in the States: the farther from the core, the better the address. After 1945, developers built millions of suburban houses, ball fields, strip malls, and office parks, effectively printing their own money as they did so. Between 1950 and 1970, the suburban population doubled from thirty-seven million to seventy-four million as an area the size of Rhode Island was developed annually.[1]

Prewar America had been quintessentially urban. Immigrants stuffed

1. Is it a mere coincidence that so many occurrences, both man-made and natural, are conveniently Rhode Island–size? Little Rhody has become a standard measure. Israel is twice the size of Rhode Island. Mountain Pine Beetles have ravaged a Rhode Island–size area of forest in Wyoming. A Rhode Island–size hole has been found in the Antarctic ice shelf.

Bobby-soxers keep hopping as the rallies fly thick and fast in this Truscon Base Coatings advertisement from October 1950.

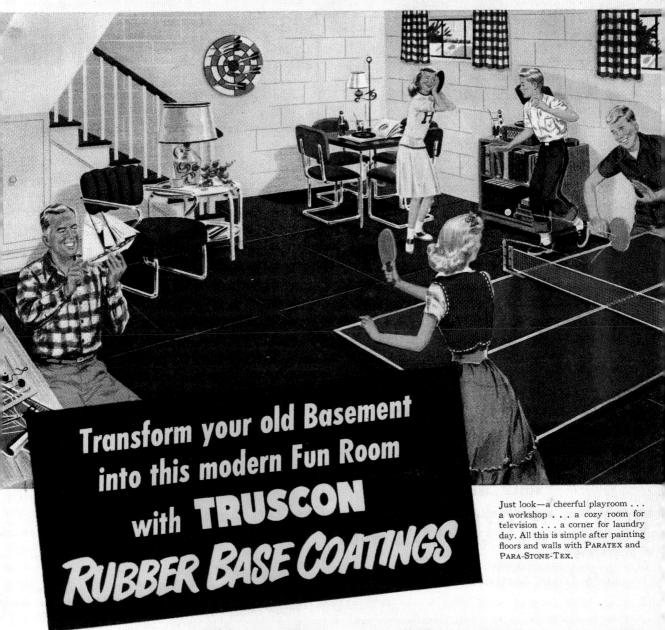

Transform your old Basement into this modern Fun Room with **TRUSCON** *Rubber Base Coatings*

Just look—a cheerful playroom . . . a workshop . . . a cozy room for television . . . a corner for laundry day. All this is simple after painting floors and walls with PARATEX and PARA-STONE-TEX.

..it's easy with *ParaTex* and *Para-Stone-Tex*

RUBBER BASE FLOOR AND MASONRY COATINGS!

MAYBE you've always shied away from modernizing your basement. Too much trouble and too expensive, you've thought.

Or maybe you had no success with *ordinary* paints—which can't "stand up" on masonry surfaces because of destructive alkali conditions always found in cement.

BUT— with PARATEX Rubber Base Floor Coating and PARA-STONE-TEX for walls, it's a different story. These wonderful rubber-base coatings resist alkali in concrete and masonry surfaces. *They're especially made for basements!* You see—the base in these coatings is a rubber resin *which is not softened by alkali.*

PARATEX and PARA-STONE-TEX come in non-fading gay colors . . . exceptionally easy to put on . . . dry hard in less than a day. And for sealing a leaky basement wall use TITEWALL IRON METHOD WATERPROOFING —you do it yourself . . . takes only a few hours . . . solution soaks into wall pores . . . expands 4 times normal size to lock out all moisture with an *iron grip.*

Write Dept. C-6, Truscon Laboratories, Detroit 11, Mich., for complete information on modern fun rooms . . . it's FREE!

Visit your neighborhood paint dealer today. He'll be glad to tell you more about PARATEX and PARA-STONE-TEX.

themselves into city neighborhoods, lacing sagging washing lines across densely packed streets, with the sound of windows being smashed by errant stickballs, and the stench of body odor intermingled with cooking. In these communities, it was impossible not to poke your nose in everyone's business. Every day looked like a scene in *Godfather II*, Vito stalking the pompous Fanucci through Little Italy's Festival of San Gennaro.

How were thousands persuaded to transform their lives from the densely packed community of the urban setting into a private world of conformity and materialism? Becoming homeowners, yes, but doing so amid a sprawling, bland, conservative culture rife with fondues, gin rummy games, and kaffeeklatschs? After copious years of research, the answer becomes clear: ping pong was the lyre-wielding Siren that lured aspirational suburbanites to their doom on the rocks. Before Madison Avenue had the bright idea of delivering trucks of cash to celebrities' doorsteps to act as pitchmen, inviting Jerry Seinfeld to hawk Microsoft, Michael Jordan to flog undies, and leaving Billy Mays to hock just about everything else, beloved ping pong was recruited to sell America on modern notions of the good life.

The great challenge facing those early Mad Men was the crushing uniformity and repetition of those suburbs, the centerless rows of ranch houses and colonials, bereft of community. External photographs were not useful advertisements for the simple reason that everything looked the same—yard after yard, garage after garage, as far as the eye could see. But in agencies across the land the solution was soon discovered: leveraging the innocence of ping pong. If the American way of life was to be tied to the notion that every man shall have his space, few things said space and freedom more than the hardwood paneling of your own finished basement—a room no one had in the big city. And what glorified that underground wonderland better than a self-contained athletic arena? And so the romance of ping pong was used to promote the image of prosperity, happiness, and family togetherness, persuading urban dwellers to migrate to the sprawling, featureless world of the subdivisions like wildebeest traversing the Serengeti. Simply put, to possess a ping pong table was to own a piece of the American dream. To quote and improve the

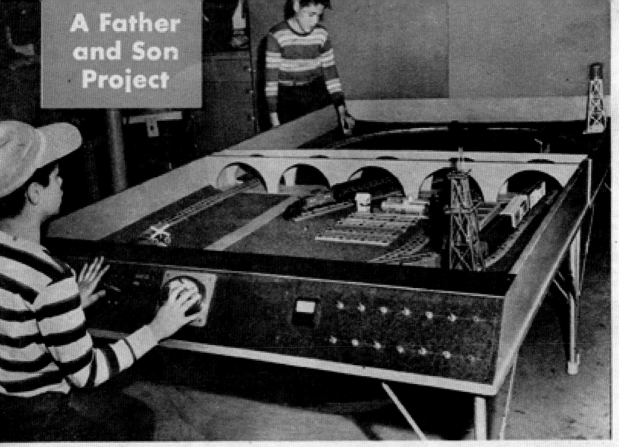

The finished combination table. The two playing surfaces for Ping Pong are in background.

Table Tennis Railroad Pike

Not sure which suburban staple should dominate your finished basement? A train set or ping pong table? *Mechanix Illustrated* magazine lets you have your cake and eat it, too, February 1953.

quintessentially American poet Robert Frost, "Home is the place where, when you have to go there, they have to take you in . . . to play ping pong."

The resulting torrent of advertisements contains many of the elements that made postwar America great: conspicuous consumption, the invention of "leisure," freedom, family, and fun. The homes themselves were always gleaming, supported by U.S. Steel—American-made, lined with "100% Nylon Fun Carpets," accessorized by assorted deer heads, banners from colleges (either

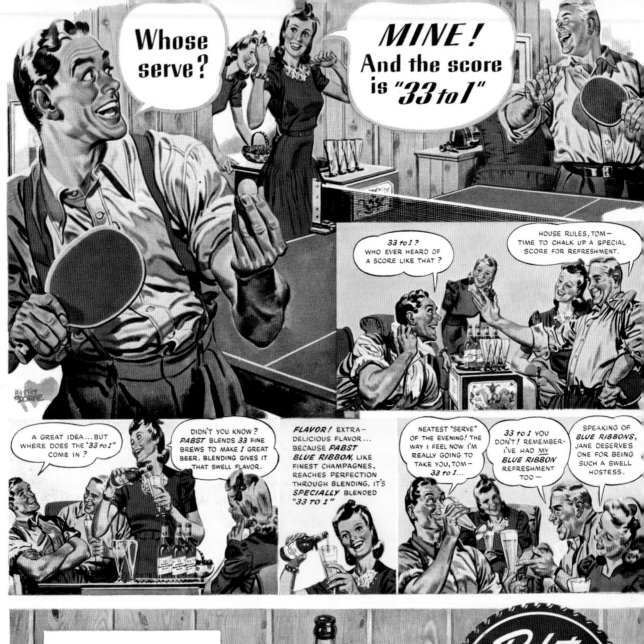
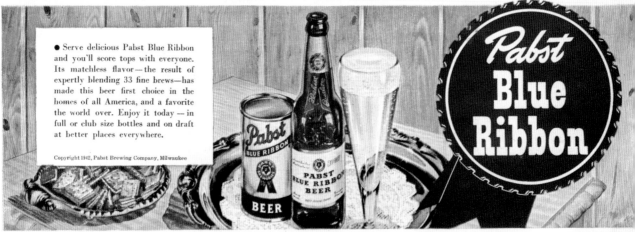

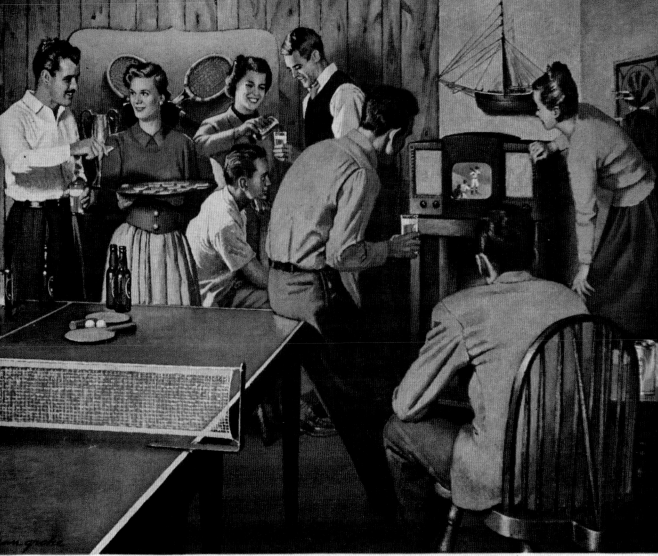

"BASEBALL ON TELEVISION," by Glenn Grohe. Number 16 in the series "Home Life in America," by noted American illustrators.

Beer belongs...enjoy it

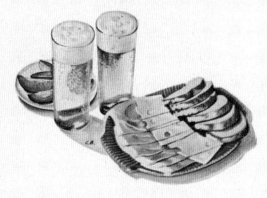

In this home-loving land of ours . . . in this America of kindliness, of friendship, of good-humored tolerance . . . perhaps no beverages are more "at home" on more occasions than good American beer and ale.

For beer is the kind of beverage Americans like. It belongs—to pleasant living, to good fellowship, to sensible moderation. And our right to enjoy it, this too belongs—to our own American heritage of personal freedom.

AMERICA'S BEVERAGE OF MODERATION

alma mater or those the kids may one day attend through osmosis), and an arsenal of landscape paintings showcasing the kind of outdoor space that lured the owners out to the suburbs in the first place.

In the giddy world of these ads, the promise of Home, the dream of Freedom, and the product to be pitched became a triptych, interchangeably connected, as in the ad for American beer: "In this home-loving land of ours . . . in this America of kindliness of Friendship, of good-humored tolerance . . . perhaps no beverages are more at home on more occasions that good American beer and ale. For beer is the kind of beverage Americans like. It belongs to pleasant living, to good fellowship, to sensible moderation. And our right to enjoy it, this too belongs—to our own American heritage of personal freedom."

The 1950s were viewed as the golden age of the American Family. The postwar marriage boom triggered a population explosion in a thousand neighborhoods named Walnut, Oak, and Paradise. Community had been left far behind in the city, but the collective that endured was the idyllic nuclear family. Dad, Mom, Buddy, and Mary are rarely happier than when playing ping pong together—which begs the question, what is the point of striking out from the dense urban conditions for the space of the suburbs if all you are going to do is hang out in the one room that has no windows? The ads also mask a reality of suburban life in which a hive of specialized activities were on offer—sporting leagues for the kids, charitable committees for women, and men's clubs for Dad, that the entire family being together was actually a rarity, apart from gathering around the television set for whatever treacly *Father Knows Best*-esque sitcom passed as "Must See TV."

All suburban kids portrayed are pert and well behaved. The boys have a short back and sides; the girls are bobby-soxed. Everyone is skinny, despite the cases of soda and ever present towers of Jane Parker Donuts ("golden puffs of lightness") stacked in every room. Wide-eyed and innocent, these children are just a decade or so away from growing their hair long, turning on, tuning in, dropping out, and letting their freak flags fly.

Ping pong paddles at rest in the top left of the picture of this Jane Parker Donuts advertisement, circa 1950.

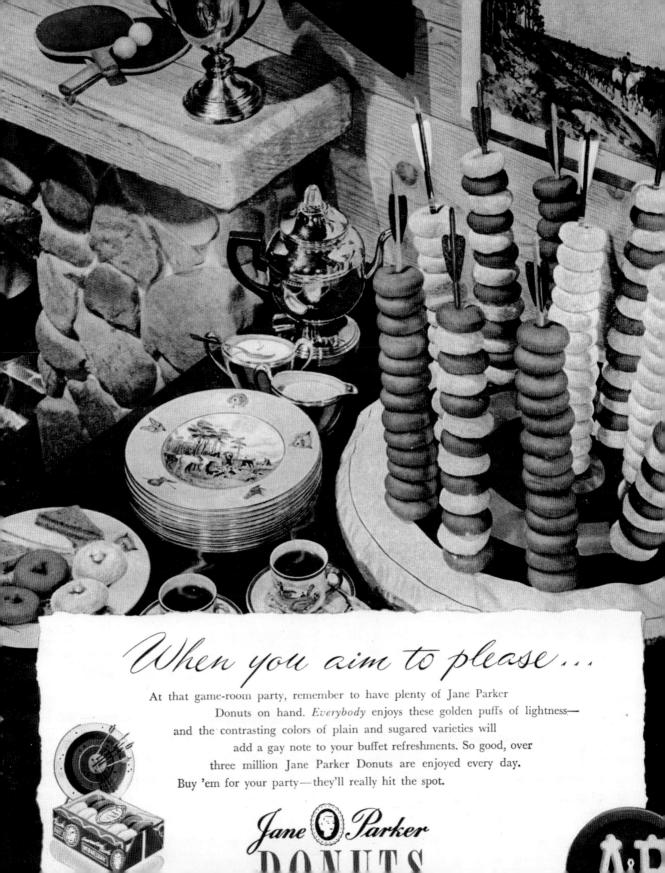

When you aim to please...

At that game-room party, remember to have plenty of Jane Parker Donuts on hand. *Everybody* enjoys these golden puffs of lightness— and the contrasting colors of plain and sugared varieties will add a gay note to your buffet refreshments. So good, over three million Jane Parker Donuts are enjoyed every day. Buy 'em for your party—they'll really hit the spot.

Jane O *Parker*

DONUTS

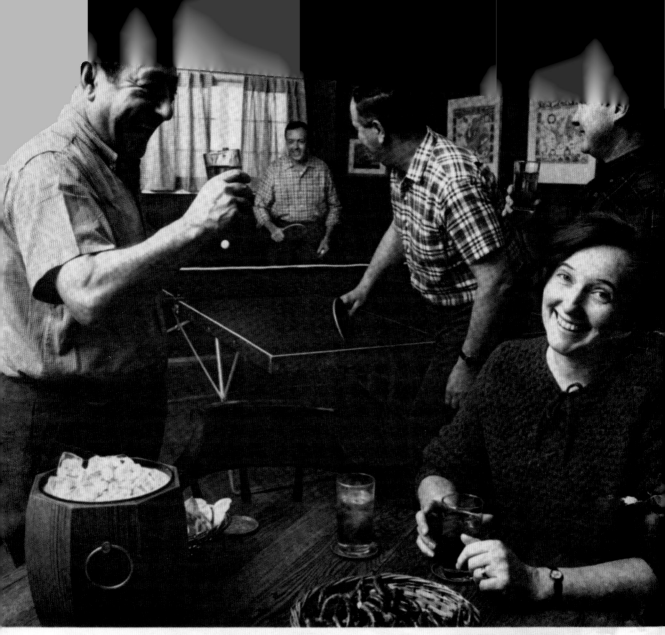

Taste is the name of the game.

That's what Imperial is all about. This rich tasting whiskey is just a sip smoother than the rest. Hiram Walker makes it that way. Game for taste? Taste Imperial. One of America's largest selling whiskeys.

Imperial

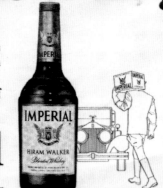

Whiskey by Hiram Walker

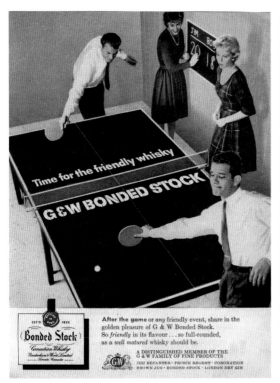

Time for the friendly whisky

G&W BONDED STOCK

After the game or *any* friendly event, share in the golden pleasure of G & W Bonded Stock. So *friendly* in its flavour . . . so full-rounded, as a *well matured* whisky should be.

A DISTINGUISHED MEMBER OF THE
G & W FAMILY OF FINE PRODUCTS

1832 DECANTER · PRINCE REGENT · CORONATION
BROWN JUG · BONDED STOCK · LONDON DRY GIN

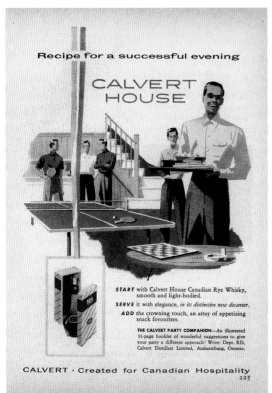

Recipe for a successful evening

CALVERT HOUSE

START with Calvert House Canadian Rye Whisky, smooth and light-bodied.

SERVE it with elegance, *in its distinctive new decanter.*

ADD the crowning touch, an array of appetizing snack favourites.

THE CALVERT PARTY COMPANION—An illustrated 32-page booklet of wonderful suggestions to give your party a different approach! Write: Dept. RD, Calvert Distillers Limited, Amherstburg, Ontario.

CALVERT · Created for Canadian Hospitality

225

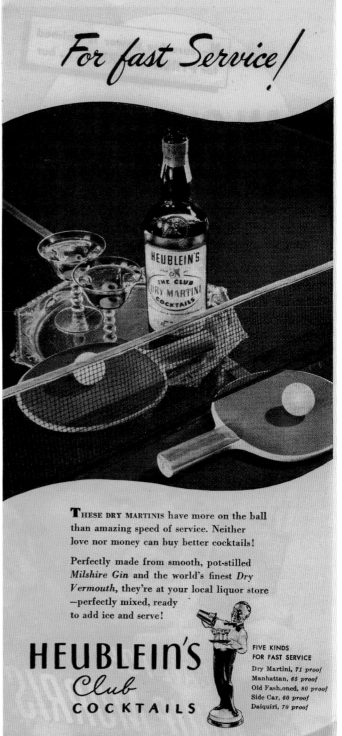

For fast Service!

THESE DRY MARTINIS have more on the ball than amazing speed of service. Neither love nor money can buy better cocktails!

Perfectly made from smooth, pot-stilled *Milshire Gin* and the world's finest *Dry Vermouth*, they're at your local liquor store —perfectly mixed, ready to add ice and serve!

HEUBLEIN'S Club COCKTAILS

FIVE KINDS
FOR FAST SERVICE

Dry Martini, *71 proof*
Manhattan, *65 proof*
Old Fash.oned, *80 proof*
Side Car, *60 proof*
Daiquiri, *70 proof*

Milshire Distilled London Dry Gin is 90 proof, distilled from 100% grain neutral spirits. G. F. Heublein & Bro., Inc., Hartford, Conn.

Left: Imperial Whiskey advertisement by Hiram Walker in 1969. *Above:* Liquor and ping pong, three advertisements from 1949 to 1969 showcasing men at play.

Dad is a career man, the epitome of virility with hair Brylcreemed to per-fection. Although the entire family lives by his success in the workplace, and dies by his failure, he manages to spend a fair amount of time at home honing his topspin backhand serve—snatching a quick game with the kids after work, or a more serious session with the guys late at night. After donning a short-sleeved check shirt, a uniform connoting leisure time, many an evening is spent in the company of men, compensating for the loss of community by organizing nights of competitive ping pong, with the sweat washed away by the beers, scotches, or martinis (which boast "more on the ball than amazing speed of service") guzzled by the dozen.

Herbert Gans's groundbreaking sociological studies of life in 1960s Levittown, New Jersey, uncovered that the move to the suburbs was trans-formational enough to improve married life, though only temporarily. For a short burst of time, fathers found happiness in home improvement, eager to tinker around the house, searching for ways to add value—for example, by converting a train set into a ping pong table by making light work of the com-plex instructions in *Mechanix Illustrated* magazine. This sense that the nest could never be feathered enough saw corner stores replaced by their big-box successors, driven by purchasing power, low prices, and an insatiable hunger to transform old basements into "modern fun rooms." Happiness was in. Old was passé. Unfortunately, the domestic bliss couldn't last; paints fresh out of the Truscon Laboratory may have come in "nonfading gay colors," but they were unable to prevent the divorce rate's soaring in the 1960s.

If Dad's place was the office, Mom was a creature of the home. Indeed, her job was the house itself, as the notion of a "housewife" entered common par-lance. Women were there to nurture, tidy, make finger sandwiches, and gen-erally service the fun that everyone else was having. More women attended college in the 1920s than in the 1950s; the modern mom was too busy for all of that. Her sense of self was expressed through shopping and homemaking. To market their products, advertisers tapped into her hopes and fears, and so a mother is visible in almost every shot, arriving in the nick of time to serve ample refreshments or to clean up a mess, her valor protected by an apron.

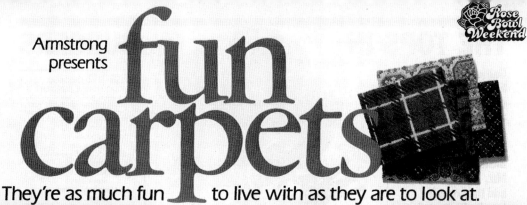

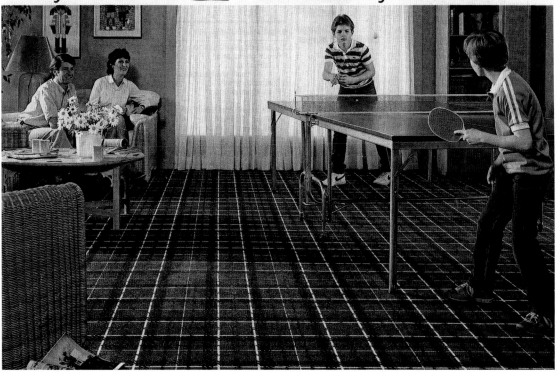

Our money is on the kid in the Nike Penetrators. An ad for Armstrong fun carpets, circa 1983.

Never has household drudgery looked so fun. In truth, boredom, loneliness, and depression predominated—what Betty Friedan referred to as the "problem with no name" in her revolutionary 1963 manifesto *The Feminine Mystique*. Freidan exposed the reality of women gripped by a sense that life had more to offer than just another child, a new recipe, or a trip to the hairdresser. The book sold over a million copies, triggering feminism's second wave.

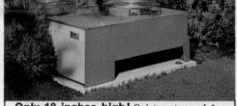

Only 18 inches high! Quiet motor and fan reduce sound; upward air discharge protects home and shrubbery.

York's new whole-house air conditioner runs so smoothly, so quietly, your neighbors will never <u>hear</u> how comfortable you are!

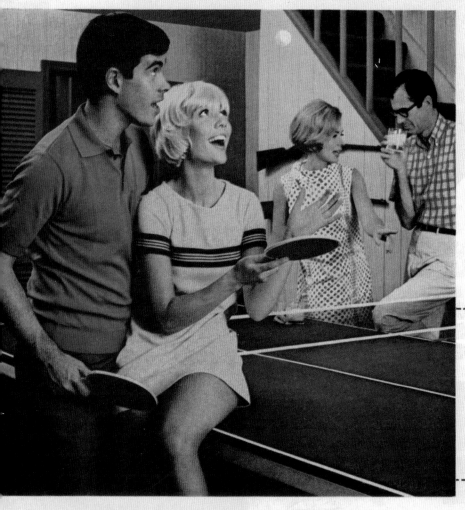

Now you can enjoy whole-house comfort conditioning without making a big noise about it! York has found a *quiet* way to air condition your home—with an advanced system that gives you full cooling power in a modern, compact package. Moving parts are isolated in a "sound deadening chamber." The powerful motor and fan run slowly, quietly. All this in a beautiful unit that's only 18 inches high!

So if you've been putting off air conditioning your home, act now—because York has built the high-performance system that assures quiet, dependable cooling and dehumidifying for any home, with any kind of heating system.

***A better way to
make you feel better***

- -

FREE AIR CONDITIONING ANALYSIS!

YORK AIR CONDITIONING
York, Pennsylvania 17405

Yes, I'd like information on York's free air conditioning analysis, and convenient monthly payment plan for homeowners.

NAME

ADDRESS

CITY

STATE   ZIP

TELEPHONE NO.   L6218

YORK
DIVISION OF BORG-WARNER CORPORATION

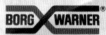

Notably missing from these ads is a dose of color. They collectively rein-forced the myth of ethnic homogeneity that existed in the suburbs. In real-ity, African Americans were part of the urban exodus, in both mixed suburbs such as New Rochelle, New York, and Montclair, New Jersey, and in all-black suburbs like Webster Groves, Missouri; Robbins, Illinois; or Glenarden, Maryland. By 1960, 2.5 million African Americans were living the suburban life, but they were written out of the telling by marketers. The mix of blue-collar class and race did not make for great ad copy.

And so, the basement ping pong table became a nation's happy place, or at least a calming urban womb grafted onto the cold reality of the American suburb. The question must be asked: What impact did the widespread prolifer-ation of ping pong tables actually have on the standard of the North American game? Canadian national coach Tony Kiesenhofer has been a proponent of the theory that suburbia weakened North American ping pong and that big houses were to blame. Those houses "large enough to store a table in a basement or a garage mean that the encounter with ping pong happens in-formally . . . Asia's more compact domestic spaces mean kids play at a sports club where they will also begin to be trained and organized." If Kiesenhofer is right—and who are we to question the depth of his spatial analysis?—then we should prepare ourselves for a ping pong renaissance. The 2008 census in-dicated that our nation's cities are experiencing a resurgence as the recession, a slump in the housing market, and higher gas prices have altered migration patterns. As New York, Chicago, and Los Angeles experience record down-town growth, expect an uptick in our nation's ping pong performance. After all, just try and fit a table in your downtown pied-à-terre.

Sun, Sea, and Spin

Once the war-era ration books had been put away, they were quickly forgotten and replaced in the 1950s by a magical time of plenty: gasoline ranneth free, highways unfurled their asphalt paths of promise, and the notion of vacationing was introduced to the masses. Luxurious resorts and gussied-up motels cluttered the landscape, fighting to cater for every price point as prosperity showered its intoxicating good fortune on every Tom, Dick, and Harry; one and all hit the road in search of the carefree fun that could only be experienced on a family vacation.

Despite *Table Tennis Magazine*'s best efforts to promote exotic trips to foreign climes—in 1951 it hailed Nigeria as the "Hottest T.T. Hotspot in the World" (noting that the "Acra team was established before Lagos and the players are mostly penholders whilst those of Lagos are of the orthodox style")—the majority of fun-seeking frolickers stayed within the borders of the continental United States, packing the kids into the car to stuff resorts from the Catskills to California. Hotel proprietors raced to distinguish themselves, luring prospective guests by promising them the world: cordon bleu cuisine, a barrage of activities, and constant entertainment. Their challenge was to find a way to deliver all of this—and keep the members of the average family away from one another's throats—without going bankrupt. Evidently the answer was almost always ping pong. Tables were ordered by the dozen, offering multigenerational fun in all weathers, indoors and out.

The phenomenon was not restricted to American shores. Butlin's, the holiday camps beloved by British working-class vacationers, constructed a psychedelic barn packed with tables as far as the eye could see, yet demand evidently ran so high they added warning signs urging PLEASE LIMIT YOUR PLAY TO 10 MINUTES IF OTHERS ARE WAITING.

The marriage of vacation and ping pong spawned a number of sporting inventions. The compact power of the ping pong Speedo was on display at New York's Napanoch Country Club, as one handsome muscleman shamelessly rallied stripped down to his bare essentials. Brilliant minds at the Pocono Mountains "Inn in the Sky" tweaked ping pong convention to conjure the "new sensational-looking game of SMASH." The outcome was the same in both cases. The Napanoch Man-kini attracted a flotilla of lilo-borne spectators who surreptitiously inched nearer to steal a glance at his fetching equipment. Similarly, the radical excitement of SMASH was a standing-room-only activity. On vacation, watching ping pong was the only thing that trumped playing it.

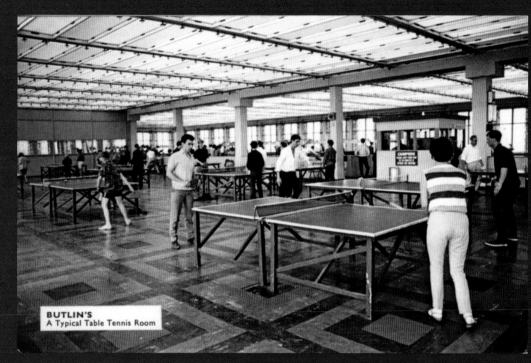

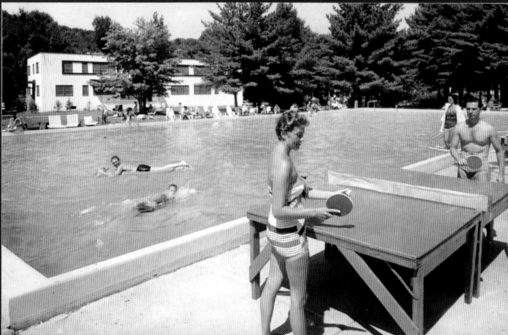

Top: Butlin's table tennis room, stamped Essex, July 1970.
Bottom: Ping Pong Speedo on display at the Napanoch

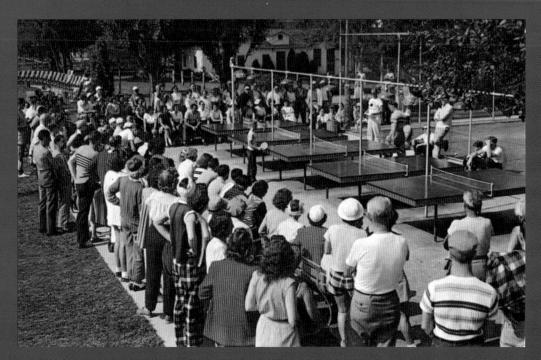

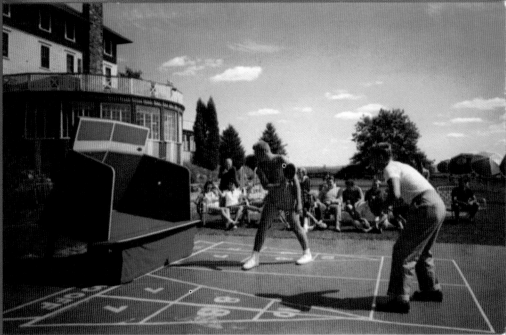

Top: "Ping pong tournament at the Sugar Maples Resort, Maplecrest-in-the-Catskills."
Bottom: "SMASH! Another first for P.M.I. in the Sky at the Pocono Mountains Inn and Cozy Cottages, Cresco 17, Pennsylvania."

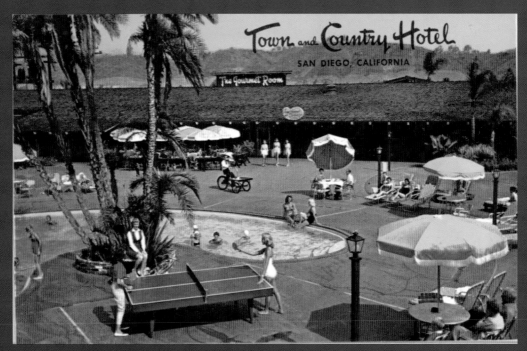

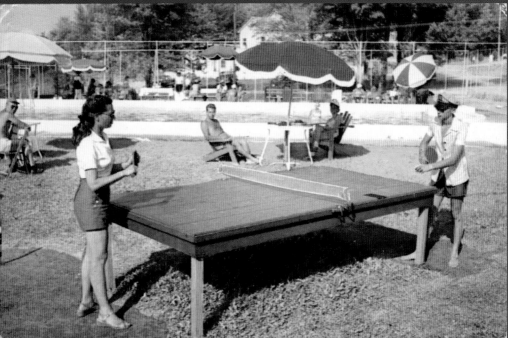

Top: "Town and Country Hotel, San Diego, California."
Bottom: "Western View Hotel, Ulster Heights-Ellenville, New York."

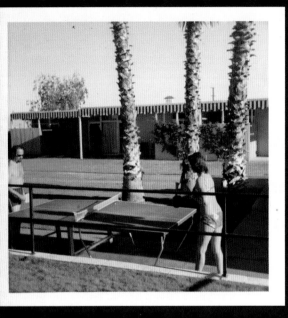

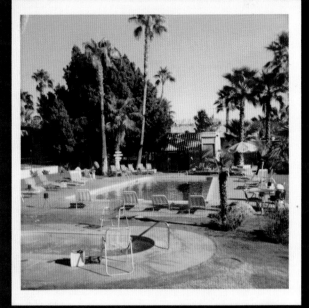

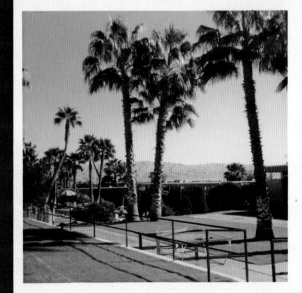

Three west coast vacation scenes, circa late 1950s.

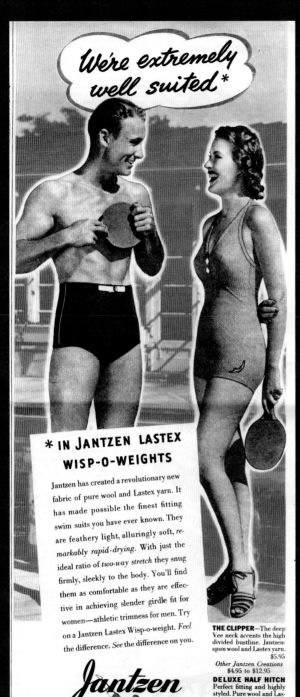
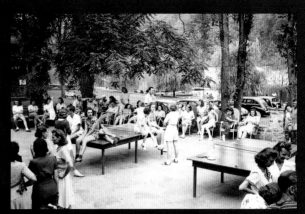

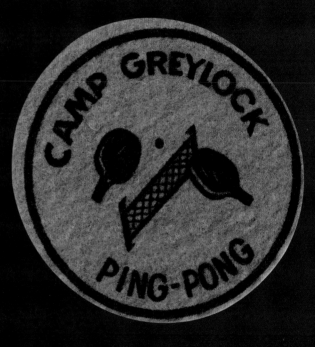

CAMP GREYLOCK
PING-PONG

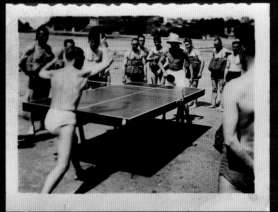

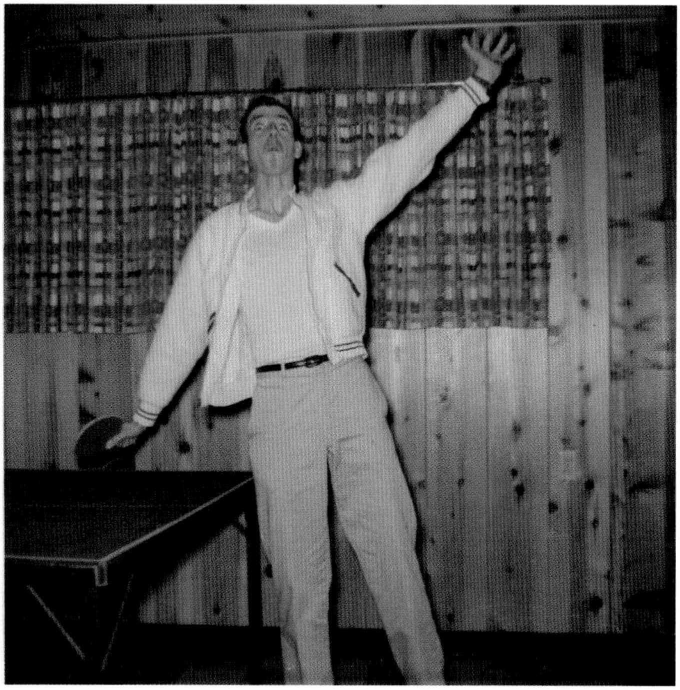

THOUGHTS FROM HOME

BY JONATHAN SAFRAN FOER

Birds do not sing, they communicate.
Humans are the only animals that sing. Or play ping pong.

It is a mistake to think about where your shot will go.
But it is a mistake not to think about it, also.

Not all of the dead are former ping pong players,
but all former ping pong players are dead.

Ping pong is to masturbation as masturbation is to sex.
Ping pong is sex without someone else and without yourself.

It is only from the top of the tallest building in the city that one can
avoid seeing the tallest building in the city.
It is only when playing ping pong that you are not there.

To rhyme words on a page is not to write poetry.
To hit a ping pong ball across a ping pong table
with ping pong rackets is not to play ping pong.

The student asks, "Why should I hit with spin?" The teacher says,
"Because you cannot spin the universe around the ball."

A serve is not a way of starting a point, but ending one.

The net is not something to be avoided like a pothole,
but approached like an asymptote.

You cannot know your limits at ping pong,
because that is one of your limits at ping pong.

One's weaknesses at the ping pong table are less remarkable than all
the things one has imagined to be one's strengths.

There is no need to apologize
when the ball hits the top of the net and falls over.
And there is no need to apologize
when a shot nicks the edge of the table
and is redirected at an impossible angle.
Only thoughtless shots need to be apologized for.
And shots derived from thought.

Despair says, *I cannot hit with the speed of my opponent*.
Happiness says, *I do not need to.*

I couldn't convince my opponent that I came in peace,
so I had to destroy him.

Pity the ping pong player who knows everything,
for he has to fear surprise.

Only the dead have discovered what they cannot live without.
It is probably ping pong.

Loving your opponent takes away his right to hate you.
It is kinder to endure being the enemy he needs.

A point is only a point, but a match is only a match.

Experience teaches the ping pong player
what won't ever happen,
which is nothing.

At the moment of the serve, the point is entirely unknowable.
But as it happens, it begins to seem explainable.
Once it is over, it could not have happened otherwise.
Next point.

All the falling rain is caught.
Every shot hits something.

Clouds keep the sun from our eyes.
Low ceilings prevent lobs.

No shot is more real than the impossible shot.

As a child I wanted to be right about my ping pong abilities.
Now I want to be wrong.

The best way to have your opponent play into your hands
is not to care about what you want him to do.

A ping pong player with one good shot has none.

I could explain how I hit my winner,
but then you would understand my explanation, not my winner.

If I didn't spend so much time playing ping pong,
I would have a much fuller life.
But I would have no life.

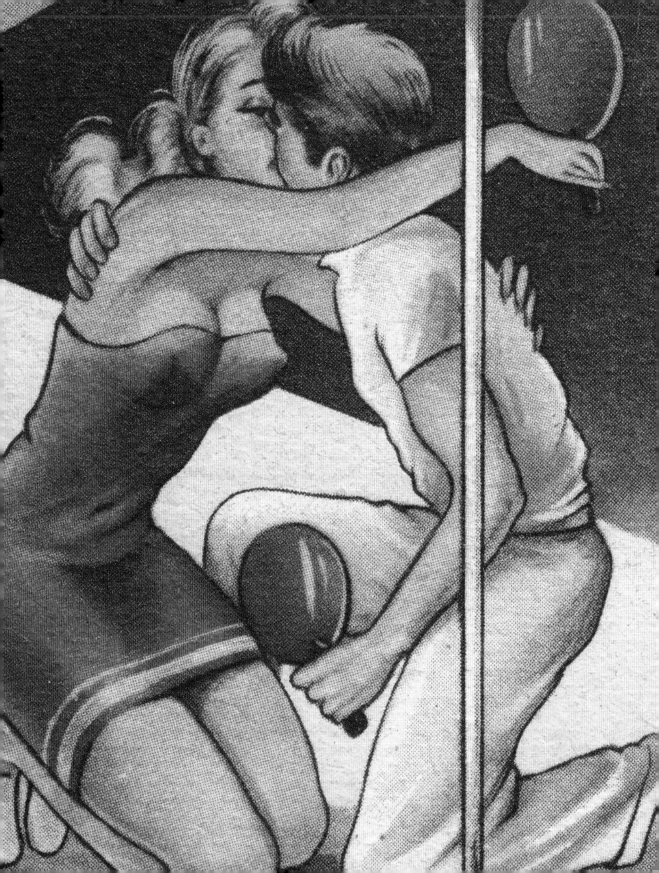

3

FOREHAND FOREPLAY

AND THE

TOPSPIN SEDUCTION

PING PONG AS APHRODISIAC

The spins. The slams. The serves, the fakes, the mistakes. The rubber paddles. The harder you hit, the harder it comes back at you, and sometimes luck is more important than skill. This is what we talk about when we talk about love.

Wiser men than I have described an intense ping pong match as a dance, and that may be true. But this dance is no restrained ballet, no genteel foxtrot. Nay, ping pong at its finest is a tango, an erotic tussle that leaves both players mussed and the paddles moist. The game contains multitudes, but at its core is an intimate pair (or, sometimes, a foursome). Ping pong is love, and love is ping pong.

This pastime gives us a language for the twists and turns, the volleys and bounces of seduction. I ask her out: serve. She agrees: return. We go out for dinner: backhand to the corner. She inquires about my infamous "intimacy issues": short chop. I excuse myself, curl up on the bathroom floor, and tremble until she leaves the restaurant: topspin slam! Horowitz wins again. Courtship is a game of semiotics, and ping pong provides a satchel of semaphore flags. The double entendres are overdetermined, almost to the point of obscenity.

Case in point: page 109 of Coleman Clark's 1933 masterwork *Modern Ping Pong*:

> Don't aim your serves constantly to one spot. Hit two or three diagonally across the table, then place one straight down the side. Strike to the corners a few times, then one directly at your adversary. This is often his most vulnerable spot. Frequently change your position behind the table and use both forehand and backhand. Experiment—try everything.

Postcard, Kansas, 1908.

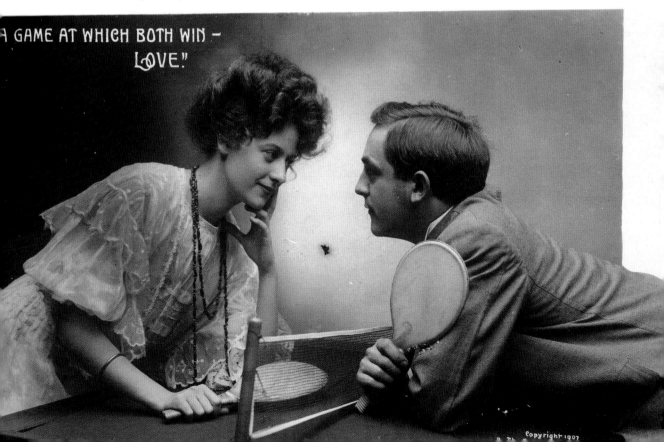

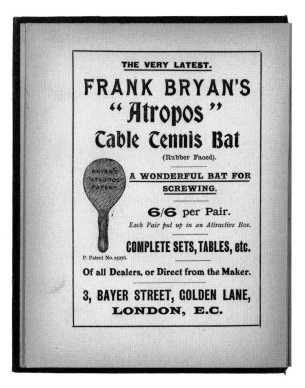

"A wonderful bat for screwing": Frank Bryan's 1901 invention of a rubbered bat opened the gates to a new era of spins.

Purr this passage to a special friend in front of a roaring fire, and watch as all proximate pants evaporate in a mist of passion. (Of course, you need to choose your page wisely; page 68, for example, might not deliver the same results: "Ping pong teaches self reliance and individual initiative and is especially recommended for boys and girls who incline toward awkwardness or who may be afflicted with inferiority complexes. . . . What an opportunity it affords them to play a game with their fathers and mothers.")

But ping pong is not just a metaphor for the mating dance—it is the dance itself. In the bastardized romantic minefield of our modern world, there are few remaining outlets where boys and girls can express themselves and learn about each other in an environment simultaneously sweaty and safe. Roller rinks have gone the way of the dodo, but ping pong strides onward into our utopian future, providing a common ground of closeness. Men are from Mars, women from Venus—but across that net, we all circle the same sun. All

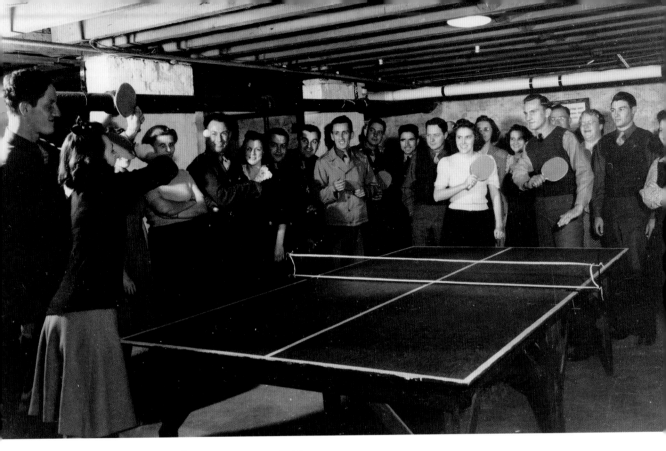

Healthy multigender interaction, circa 1960.

compete on a level table, and anyone can win, regardless of gender, preference, or body type. And we're not talking about some limp party game, some witty banter across a Scattergories board. This is flailing limbs, dancing feet, and a healthy dose of steely competition—a pretty close simulacrum of a long-term loving relationship. Ping pong offers us this terrarium, this biodome, a medium far more expressive than the text-message alternatives.

Affection depends on this communication and proximity, but seduction demands separation, a sprinkling of erotic restraint. We must be close enough to lock sexy eyes, trade sexy quips, waft sexy scents—but not so close that the quivers are quashed. As Freud wrote, "Some obstacle is necessary to swell the tide of libido to its height; and at all periods of history whenever natural barriers in the way of satisfaction have not sufficed, mankind has erected

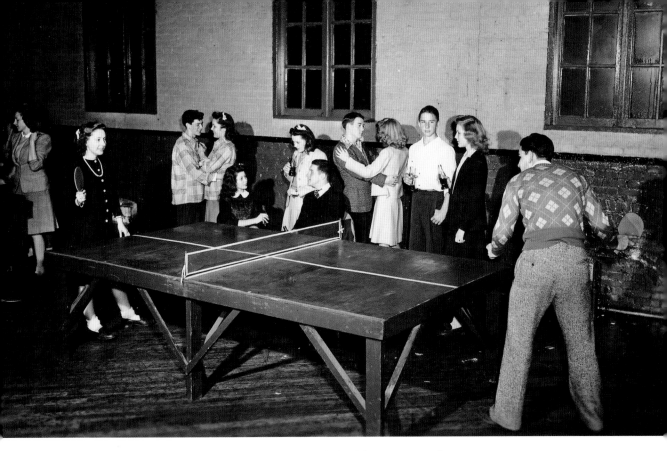

An Alabaman youth club captured halfway through the delicate transition from competition to cooperation.

conventional ones in order to enjoy love." This obstacle is ping pong's gift to eros! In our age of wanton touching and easy feeling, there's only one natural barrier remaining: those forty square feet of green particleboard (plus sixty inches of netting). No other pastime provides this precise balance, this delicate distance. Except maybe Battleship.

But Battleship doesn't make the heart go pitter-patter. And pitter-patter the heart must! Quite literally, it turns out. The classic Capilano Bridge experiment (Dutton & Aron, 1974) interviewed subjects walking across two different bridges: one narrow, wooden, swaying, and the other a sturdier modern structure. The interviews themselves were a ruse; the real data was that the men interviewed on the rickety bridge were *nine times* more likely to subsequently call the interviewer—a healthy young woman of pleasing proportions—to "discuss the experiment" (and, ya know, maybe dinner some-time?). The psychologists' conclusion was this: subjects in a state of high anxi-ety or excitement—in this case, walking on a narrow wooden bridge above a deep gorge—are far more receptive to romantic advances. The physical symp-toms of stress were subconsciously interpreted as signals of arousal, and the starry-eyed subjects responded accordingly. In other words, a quickened pulse is not a result of seduction, but rather seduction is the result of a quickened pulse. Depending on your school of interpersonal-attraction thought, this is described as misattribution, excitation transfer, or response facilitation, but the lesson is the same. A long rally ends, and there she stands—heart pound-ing, sweat-beaded, lungs heaving.[1]

Thus we find the preconditions for love: proximity, enforced separation, and preexisting physical excitement. Ping pong might not be the *only* activity that combines all three. Air hockey, perhaps. But it is certainly the only activity that combines all three plus Biljana Golic. (See page 109 for more on Ms. Golic.)

This aphrodisiac cocktail packs a punch even at the highest levels of the sport. In 2004, shortly before the Athens Olympics, four players were sent home from the Chinese table tennis team for "engaging in romantic affairs" with other players. These players knew the punishment that awaited them, and yet they still could not resist. Such is the allure of a well-gripped paddle! And these particular paddles were well gripped indeed: two of the players punished were the lady friends of the number one and two ranked men's play-ers in the world, Wang Hao and Ma Lin. (The men were not disciplined for their role in the relationships.)

But here's where it gets interesting. Not only is ping pong fertile soil for blossoming love, but the reverse is equally true as well: sexy feelings breed star paddlers. And when those feelings go unsexy, the paddlers go unstarry. These two ostracized women, Fan Ying and Bai Yang, continued to play competitive

1. Beyond the psychophysiology, there are also cosmetic benefits to this activity, as described by Pinkie Barnes in the October 1951 issue of *Table Tennis*: "The basis of all good looks is a clear, spotless skin, and there's nothing like the vigorous exercise of T.T. to help remove impurities from the skin. . . . Incidentally, I'm all for using a little rouge. You don't often start to color up until the end of the first set and it's first impressions that count."

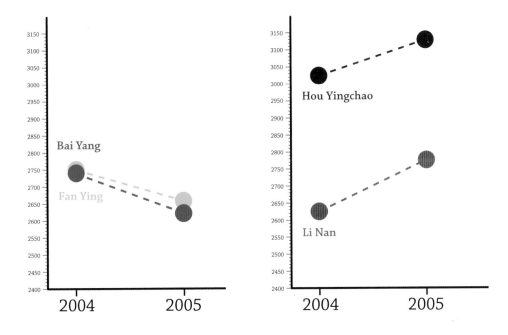

Bai's and Fan's post-breakup decline (left) contrasted with Li's and Hou's romantic getaway (right).

ping pong—but without love, their smashes had no . . . smash. In both cases, the players' ITTF rankings dropped precipitously after the 2004 heartbreaks. Their male counterparts, unpunished by the team but battered in the heart, saw their play suffer as well; Wang was upset in the finals (by a Korean!), and Ma didn't even medal.

In contrast, observe the other two players sent packing: a couple. Li Nan and Hou Yingchao were left bereft of luxury training and nationalistic glory, but they retained a richer reward: the glory of love. Expelled together, two against the world, both Li and Hou actually *improved* after leaving the team.

Love without ping pong, ping pong without love—I suppose either is *possible,* but what's the point?[2]

2. Of course, players must be careful that a love of pong doesn't become a replacement for love itself. In a chilling passage, Marty Reisman writes, "My racket became a delicate as well as a sensuous connection between the ball and my brain. The more I used it, the more dependent I became on my racket, until I was madly in love with this incredible instrument."

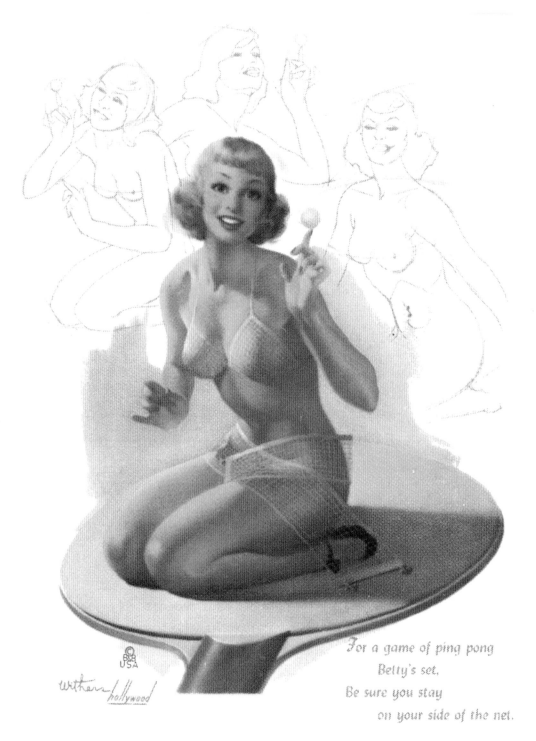

For a game of ping pong
Betty's set.
Be sure you stay
on your side of the net.

BROWN & BIGELOW
Remembrance Advertising

The first person to truly comprehend this special symmetry was Henry Miller, preeminent erotic scribe of the twentieth century. This legendary penman was also a legendary paddle-holder, famous for his ping pong passions. Even today, the Henry Miller Library in Big Sur features a table, available for play by any stoppers-by. For Miller, ping pong was not a mere pastime, a diversion from his regular life. Nay, the ball and paddle were at the core of his existence. When asked what kept him so youthful into his geriatric years, Miller replied, "The purity of my soul, playing ping pong, and above all, love!" He might as well have said, "Ping pong, playing ping pong, and above all, ping pong"—for ping pong is purity, and ping pong is love. His fountain of youth bubbled on throughout his eighth decade: across a ping pong table at a Hollywood party, he met Hoki Tokuda, forty-seven years his junior. Within months Tokuda became Miller's fifth wife; the marriage ceremony took place between two fast-paced games.

If anything else needs to be said on the special relationship between acts of pong and acts of love, we will leave it to Miller himself: "The importance of this recreation lies in preventing intellectual discussions."

Of course, it must be admitted that ping pong isn't *always* sexy. For example:

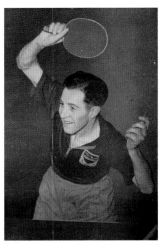

But what exactly is the problem here? The stance looks correct. The grip seems to be fundamentally sound. The pants are appropriately snug. But yet the overall effect is strangely unarousing. What is wrong with this picture?

Clearly there are possible pitfalls when attempting to harness the seductive powers of pong—and clearly that pit can fall down deep. How to avoid those dangers? What can one do to maximize one's mojo? What can *I* do to maximize *my* mojo?

This calls for an expert. By general consensus, the most important work on romantic attraction of the past eighty years is *The Art of Seduction*, by Robert Greene. Greene is the author of several other seminal works, including *The 48 Laws of Power* ("An inspiration from somewhere else" —Stephon Marbury), and *The 50th Law* (coauthored by 50 Cent). *The New Yorker* has described Greene as "a kind of sage." Surely a man inspiring such diverse praise would possess the wisdom necessary to extract the secrets of ping pong seduction. But would his theories stand up to the slams and spins of real competition? In the interests of scientific rigor and personal procreation, I decided to test them myself.

Armed with Greene's pinkish tome, I left my desk and boldly descended the stairs to the basement, where two pleasant sights awaited me: a verdant table, net tautly astrung, and a young lady, paddle in hand. We greeted each other warmly, with raised eyebrows and tentative smiles. Greene had already instructed me to Isolate the Victim: "Lure the seduced into your lair, where nothing is familiar." Done; the basement was empty, as basements often are, and there would be no doubles matches at this early point in our relationship. The paddle-wielding flower—let's call her Bethany—waggled her paddle insouciantly in my direction, and warm-ups began.

I flipped ahead to Chapter 2: Create a False Sense of Security—Approach Indirectly. This casual volleying may precede any official score keeping, but that doesn't mean there is nothing to be won or lost. In fact, the warm-ups are as important as the game itself—the bow before the dance, the flirting before the affair. I kept it easy, even, friendly; Bethany did the same. Back and forth, back and forth, we were united in a steady bounce of symbiosis. I appeared safe, reliable; trust bloomed in her eyes as she began to daydream of

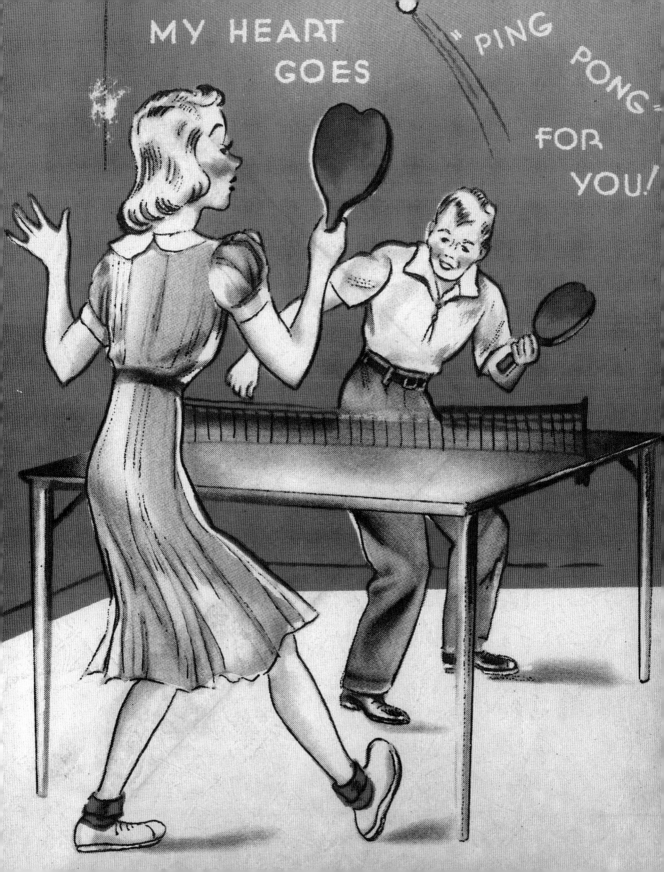

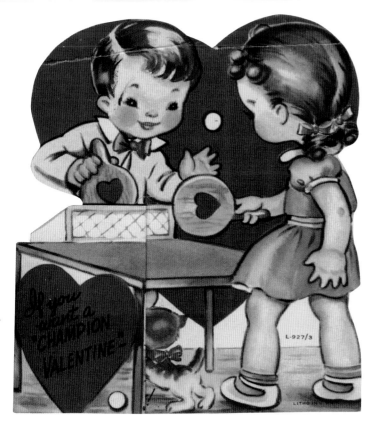

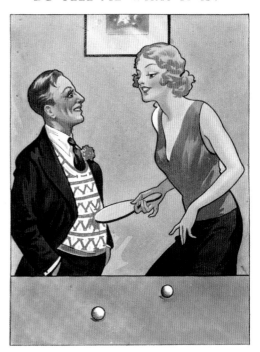

"DO YOU PLAY PING-PONG?"
"I PLAY A SHOCKING GAME."
"DO TELL ME WHAT IT IS!"

Valentines and humor cards, circa 1935–1955.

our gaggle of alliteratively named children. Oh, Bethany! Didn't your mother tell you never to give your heart to a ping pong man?

We soon were warmed. The match began.

"Poeticize your presence," says the master Greene. I attempted to play with a lyrical elegance, all sweeping forehands and piquant chops. I resisted any urge to throw my paddle. I avoided girlish yelps. My presence was iambic. My presence was Nerudian. My presence could have been read aloud by Maya Angelou. I looked across the table, at lovely Bethany. Her cheeks were flushed.

But something was not quite right. My mastery was apparent, but it was all too simple, too direct—more a business transaction than a seductive dance. I turned to Chapter 3: Send Mixed Signals. This is an area Greene discusses in great depth, and from many angles—insinuation, need, temptation—but they all can be distilled down to one daring maneuver: Lob Lob Lob Smash.

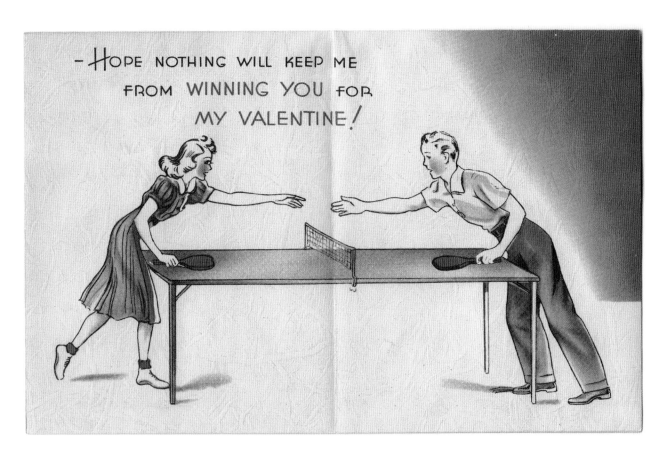

This begins with a steady sequence of high, looping shots, insinuating my way into an easy exchange, an extended volley. The steady rhythms become hypnotic and then addictive, thereby creating a need. But poor Bethany is torn, because another voice within her is nearly berserk with temptation: the ball is just floating there, so juicy, so hittable. . . . And just when this tension becomes unbearable, when the two competing desires seem they cannot endure any longer, I resolve it myself, with an unexpected, furious slam that skids off the table and into the far recesses of the damp basement. Point: Horowitz.

(For a different type of opponent—those with tournament-level skills or masochistic tendencies—an alternate strategy can be employed: the risky Smash Smash Smash Lob. This should be attempted only by experienced operators; dangers include pulled groins and lost matches. When performed correctly, however, the SSSL allows for all the benefits of LLLS, plus those

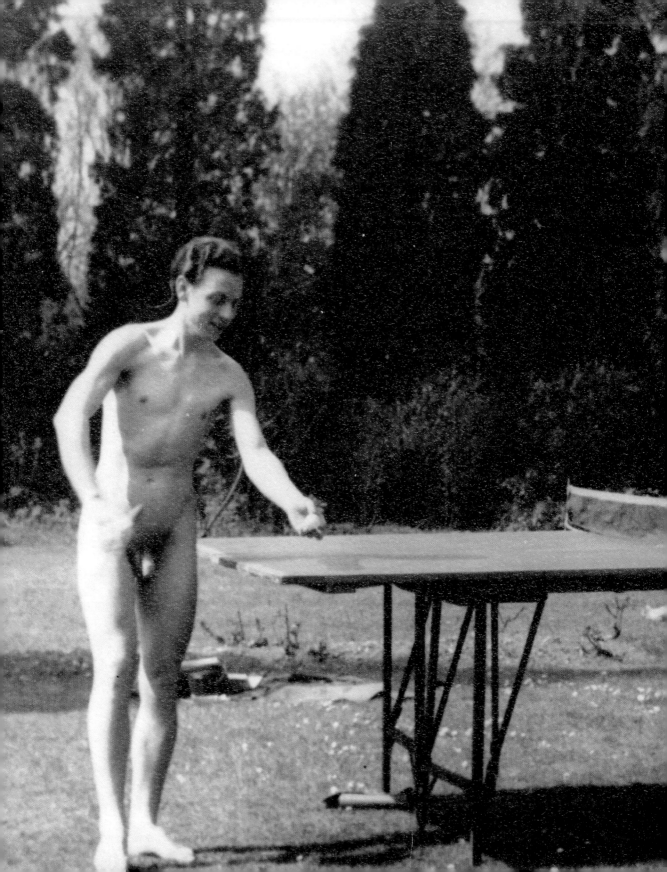

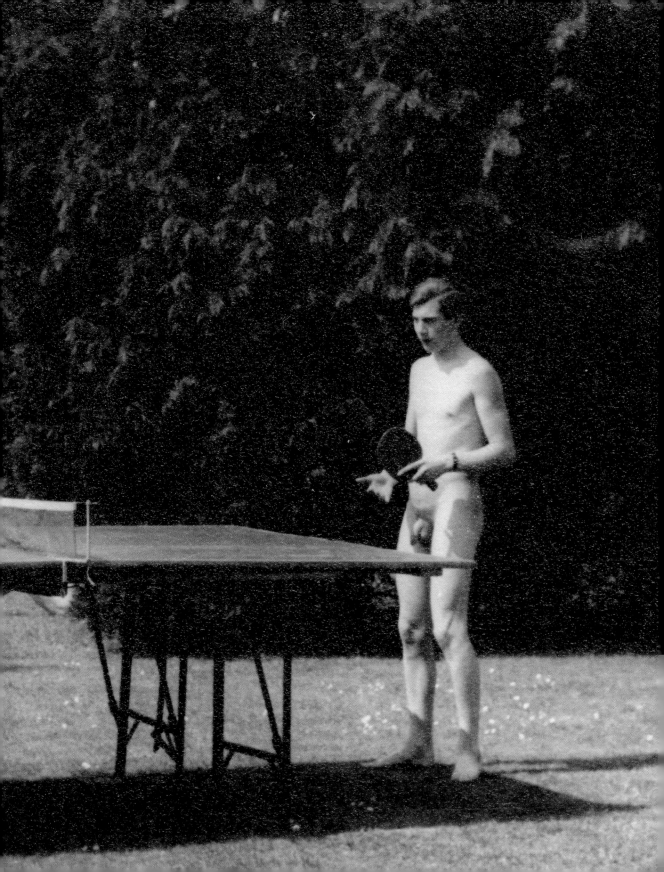

Table Tennis
Comes of Age

•

SOL SCHIFF

discussed in Chapter 21: Give Them Space to Fall—The Pursuer Is Pursued; the sweet young thing across the table gets a taste of blood, and maybe she likes it. And maybe you like it, too.)

By now, Bethany and I were deep into the match. The score was tight, and the end was near. A connection had been forged. But our rhythms, once so intoxicating, had grown a bit . . . stale. It was time for Greene's master stroke: Chapter 18: Stir Up the Transgressive and Taboo. "Master the art of the bold move," he writes. "Not everything in romantic love is supposed to be tender and soft; hint that you have a cruel, even sadistic streak." Easy for him to say; in the safety of a luxury hotel, any number of scenarios and costumes can be brought into play. But I was in a basement, facing the runaway train of Bethany's topspin slams. Various naughty options sprang to mind: switch the paddle to my other hand. Switch the paddle for a butter knife. Leap up upon the table. Remove my pants. Etc. What would Robert Greene do? What would Henry Miller do? What would Biba want? The ball crossed the net, heading my way. Time stood still. Nothing moved, except for my pounding, yearning heart.

And there we will let a veil of darkness fall over the basement. Maybe I won, maybe I lost. The important thing is to play the game; there's always another match ahead, other players in the pool. And maybe such straightforward analogies no longer apply here. Ping pong sounds like love, looks like love, works like love, and feels like love; it provides a language for describing, the physical ingredients for initiating, the emotional thrills for elevating, and the spiritual core for maintaining a lifelong affair—and yet here we are, alone again. Ping pong is love, and love is ping pong—both are eternal mysteries, and these mysteries haunt us, enchant us, sustain us.

Hits and Ass

The combination of table tennis and sex normally conjures images of Thai women, plastic balls, vaginal cavities, and pelvic muscles. But long before Viagra, when a gentleman could only rely on visual stimulation to muster wood on command, ping pong porn was often the sophisticate's choice. Sadly, this innocent genre has fallen from favor in these cruder modern times. Little is known about its origins, but we obtained the images to follow from a noted ping pong porn historian, David K. of San Francisco. David K. speculates that the genus, which thrived in still photos and on film, emerged from Southern California in the late 1960s. "The Californian dream was still on the ascent," he explains, "and ping pong pornography captured its essence. Basically, the form consisted of two innocent yet crucially well-endowed young things, typically blondes, embarking in a game of ping pong in the buff, often outdoors. Their table skills were often mediocre, but that is not why people were buying. The game's beauty lay in its ability to conjure the best out of their swaying assets."

In the film version of the genre, the two girls would rally back and forth, often playing a complete game to 21. These shoots were simple, cheap to make, and contained no naughty stuff. The thrill was voyeuristic, enhanced perhaps by subconscious memories of teen longing conjured by the ping pong action. Innocence was its strength—but also its weakness. In a world in which starlets leak sex tapes to promote their careers, the absence of explicit rumpy-pumpy led to the genre's rapid relegation to the annals of porn history. Google "Ping Pong Porn Paddle Video" if you must, for research purposes only, and you can see the tawdry, modern equivalent.

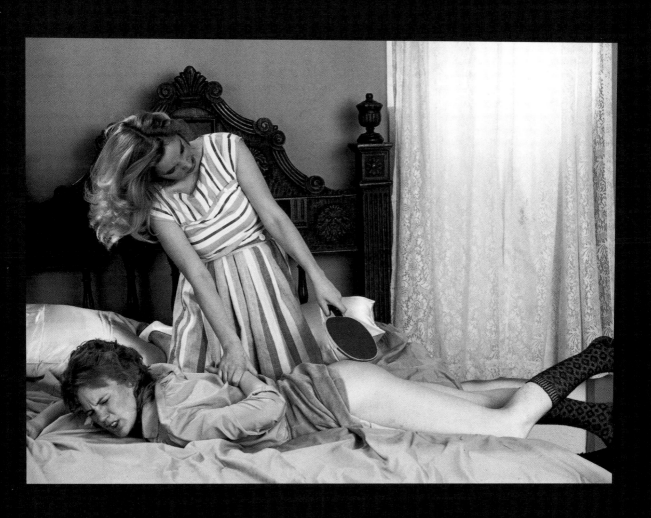

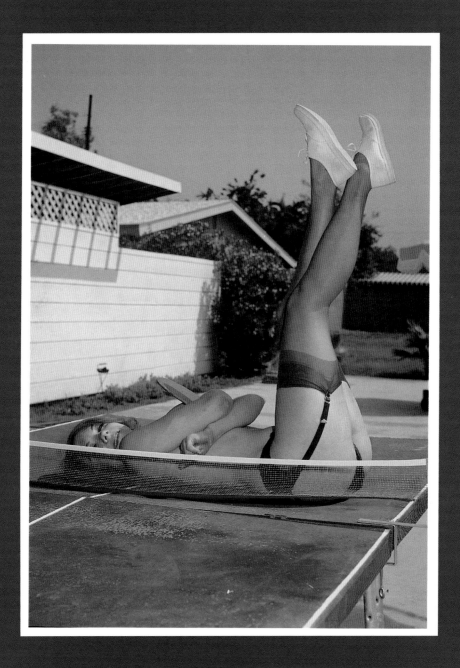

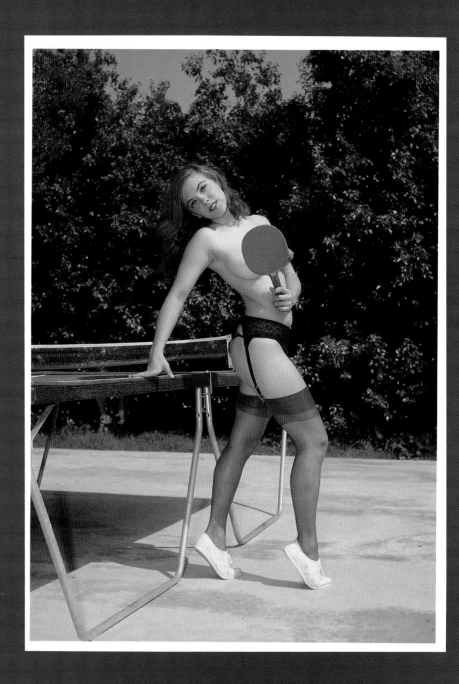

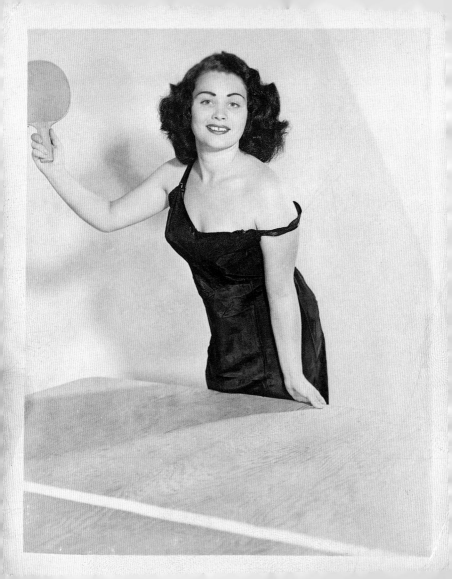

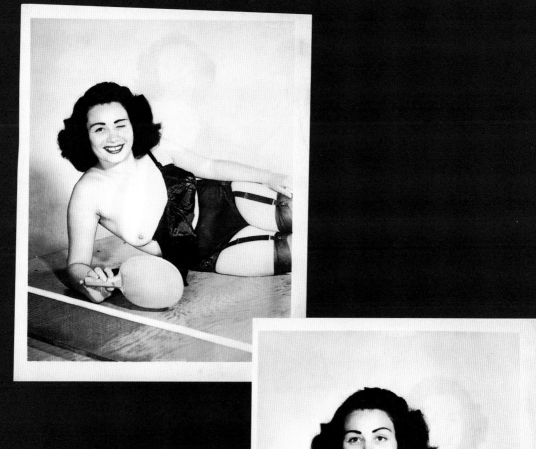
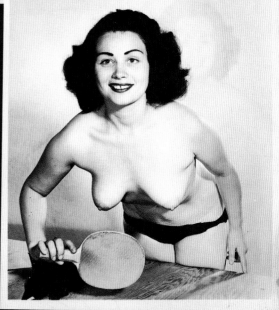

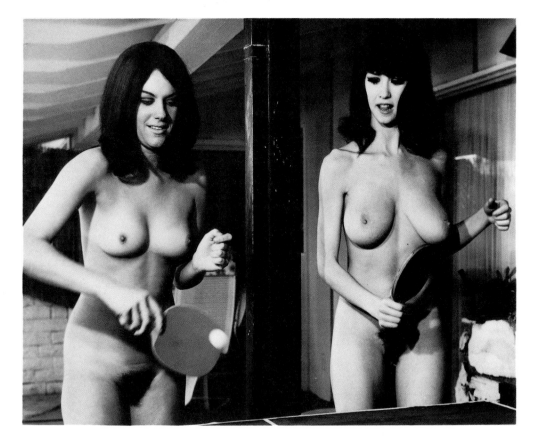

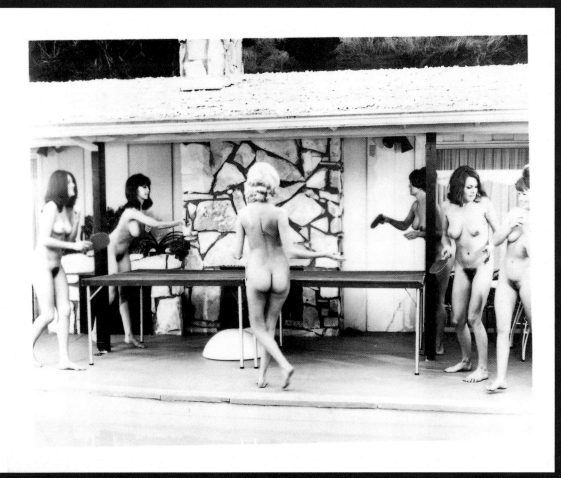

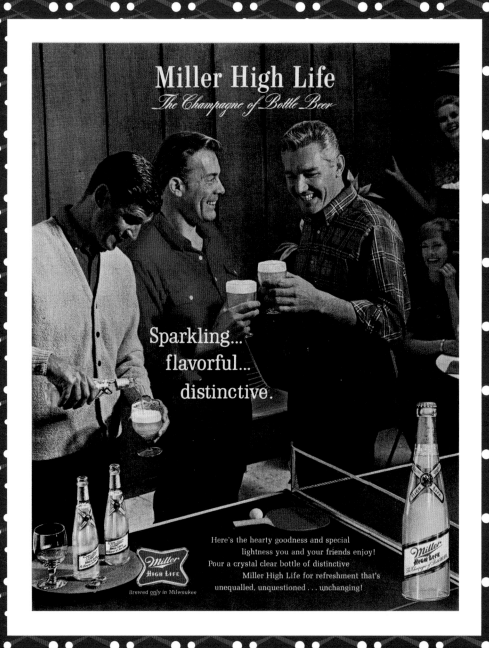

TESSA

BY DAVY ROTHBART

My cousin called the teams—me and him versus his roommate Bauer and Bauer's girlfriend, Tessa. This was down in the raw stink of a crumbling frat house basement on the Drexel University campus in West Philly. My cousin was a college junior; I was a high-school freshman, visiting town for the weekend. I'd never played beer pong before and hardly even drank.

The game, as they explained it, was simple: two plastic cups of beer perched at either end of the table. You played with paddles and everything, like regular ping pong, but if you plunked the ball against the other team's cup, both of them had to drink. Land the ball inside the cup, they had to down the whole beer. Win the game, they had to down two.

Within a half hour, we all were fucked up. Now, twenty years and a thousand drinking sessions later, I can recognize the types of drinkers each of us were. There was my cousin, the jolly, rambunctious sort of drinker who just wants to get everyone wasted, especially the shy, the officious, or the kid who's never been drunk before. That was me, the newbie who doesn't know how to measure his level of drunkenness and just keeps laughing and saying shit that doesn't make any sense, before eventually throwing up and passing out in an alleyway or on the bathroom floor. There was Bauer, the guy who turns wicked with drink, full of torn-up fury, whose only outlet is to pop someone in the eye or crack a pool cue over some poor sap's head. And then there was Tessa, the kind of beautiful girl who downs drinks in long pulls, who smiles sad smiles and plays with her jewelry and looks lost and big-eyed and at the end of the night targets a stranger to make out with to keep her seeping darkness at bay. These days I could take one fucking glance into a basement like that and tell you how shit was about to go down. But I was fifteen and I had no idea.

Bauer kept knocking over his own beers, which meant, according to house rules, that he had to drink a full cup each time as a penalty. He started shouting and swearing at us, at himself, and especially at Tessa. As my cousin and I won game after game, Bauer and Tessa got more and more drunk.

Then, for about ten minutes, they put on a surprising rally. A shot hit the net and dribbled over. Another nicked off the very end of the table, unreturnable. Before long they'd taken a 17–4 lead. Whenever they hit our cup of beer and we had to drink, I took small sips, while my cousin guzzled. "You're not drunk enough!" he roared, with an affectionate whomp on my shoulders. He explained his theory that in all sports—pool, basketball, beer pong—there was a sweet spot of drunkenness necessary to maximize your skills. Too little drink and you were tentative, indecisive; too much drink and you were popping the cue ball off the table or airballing shots over the back-board. "Down this," he said, topping off a fresh cup from the keg on the floor. I glugged the whole thing down, and Tessa clapped and smiled and flashed her green eyes at me, her beauty both painful and electrifying.

Me and my cousin immediately began an epic comeback. I found that Bauer couldn't handle the slightest bit of topspin. He howled at each point we scored, and soon his face was pink. Tessa teased an impossible shot off the corner of the table to tie the game at 19, but Bauer slapped my next serve into the net, and my cousin slammed home a drop shot to give us the win. While we celebrated with a series of emphatic high fives, Bauer and Tessa quietly drank two beers each. Bauer then mashed his empty cups against his face—one to his forehead, one to his jaw, and hauled Tessa close for a kiss on the neck. She spun away. Bauer whipped his paddle across the table; it whizzed past my ear like a throwing star and took out a chunk of wall behind my head. He lifted the entire table, crashed it onto its side, and stormed away up the stairs. Tessa stared at the table forlornly, as though it were a dying dolphin, then looked up at me and my cousin with wet eyes. In just a couple of hours, I'd fallen powerfully in love with her. I'm pretty sure my cousin was in love with her, too, but he was dating a girl up in Allentown, and he split right then to go crash at her place.

Dazed, supremely loaded, and too full of desire for Tessa to say a word to her, I found my way up to my cousin's room on the third floor of the house and sank into a bed, staring at the walls. On each wall, my cousin and Bauer had painted a giant mural representing one of Philadelphia's four major sports teams—the Phillies, the Sixers, the Flyers, and the Eagles—complete with team colors and insignias and crudely crafted faces of a few of their favorite players. They loomed over me like doctors over a sick infant—Mike Schmidt, Randall Cunningham, Moses Malone.

The door opened. Tessa slipped in. She climbed into bed beside me and without a word pressed her lips to mine. Her breath was hot, salty, and strangely coppery. For some reason, I pretended to be asleep, and then pretended to be waking from sleep. I kissed her back. My heart blammed like a tommy gun. I couldn't believe this was happening.

Tessa took hold of my hand, pressed it against her breast, and began cupping her own breast through my hand. Then she clutched my other hand—like it was a dead thing—and pushed it down her stomach and inside her jeans. "I don't have a condom," I squeaked, and she shushed me and pulled her jeans off in one deft move and tossed them into the darkness, knocking bottles off a dresser.

It was another minute or so before Bauer came crashing into the room and things turned ugly. First, though, I said to Tessa, "Wait, I just want to kiss you some more." It wasn't that I didn't want to have sex with her—I did, as badly as I'd ever wanted anything—but kissing her, just kissing her, felt so exquisite, so holy, so unimaginably thrilling, that I wanted to savor it for as long as possible. So we kissed for a few long moments, not like drunks tearing at each other, but with tenderness, longing, and real love.

A strange thing happened as we kissed—I began to replay our rounds of ping pong in my head, and suddenly all these deep truths of the game revealed themselves to me. I understood the shots I should have made, the times I'd held off the ball, waiting for my cousin to make a move when the move was mine to make, and even how I'd been balancing on my heels when I needed to shift more onto my toes. It's not that I wasn't present with Tessa, wildly in the moment with her—no, the opposite was true. I was so entirely in the moment that the whole night seemed to bleed together into one pulsing beat. Flashes from my past and from my future strobed through my mind. Everything made sense to me—where I'd been, the mistakes I'd made, and where I wanted to be and what I had to do to get there. The game and the girl were one.

It was in the midst of this that I felt my entire body jerked up-ward, like a beached whale in a chopper's sling, and then I was heaved face-first into a wall, Bauer's iron elbow pinned to my spine.

"What the fuck is going on right now?" he yelled with anguish and rage. He pulled my right arm behind my back, and my shoulder burned with pain, as though the socket might cave and let my limb loose. I opened my eyes and discovered that my face was pressed directly into the eerie portrait of Sixers point guard Maurice Cheeks. Before I could respond or even cry out, Bauer dumped me out of his room, into the stairwell, and slammed his door shut.

I faced the door; I could hear him shouting on the other side. Then he settled down, and not long after I heard him and Tessa start fucking. Hollowed, on the edge of tears, I wandered down the stairs. In the dark living room, a dozen of my cousin's housemates were passed out on sofas like victims of an atomic blast, caught in SportsCenter's grim flicker. I grabbed a stray cushion, continued on down to the basement, and sat against a wall, sipping on the last third of a beer, lost as an old-timer at the end of the bar. At last I righted the ping pong table, stretched out on top of it with the sofa cushion as a pillow, and fell fast asleep. I slipped out of the house at dawn, and a day later I was headed back to Michigan. On the train ride home I wrote Tessa a long love letter which I mailed to her parents' house in Glasgow, Delaware (the registrar's office gave me the address). I proposed that we run off together out west. I never heard back.

But it's funny the ways one night can shape you. For example, I discovered that night that ping pong tables are oddly comfortable to sleep on. I've slept on about thirty in the years since; I will always sleep on a ping pong table if the choice is between a ping pong table and the floor. Also, whenever I'm at the bar and I glance at a TV hanging from the rafters and happen to catch any Philadelphia sports highlights, I still get a strange, hot jolt—those murals in my cousin's bedroom the night I kissed Tessa, they're to credit and to blame. I'll even pass a dude on the street wearing a Phillies jersey and that room comes back to me, Mike Schmidt's bug-eyed face, the taste of Tessa's lips.

If I'd known that night, as I sat sipping the last third of a beer in the basement of my cousin's frat house, that I'd still be in love with Tessa twenty years later, that I'd be spending four nights a week at bars in cities like Mobile, Alabama, and Kansas City and Little Rock, falling in love with Tessas, dying to kiss them, would I have done anything differently? Maybe once a year I get to kiss a Tessa, the other eleven months and change I get tossed out of Bauer's room and sleep on ping pong tables, but still, if it happens even once a year, all those other nights and games are worth the trouble.

Tessa, I still love you. Tessa, see what you've done?

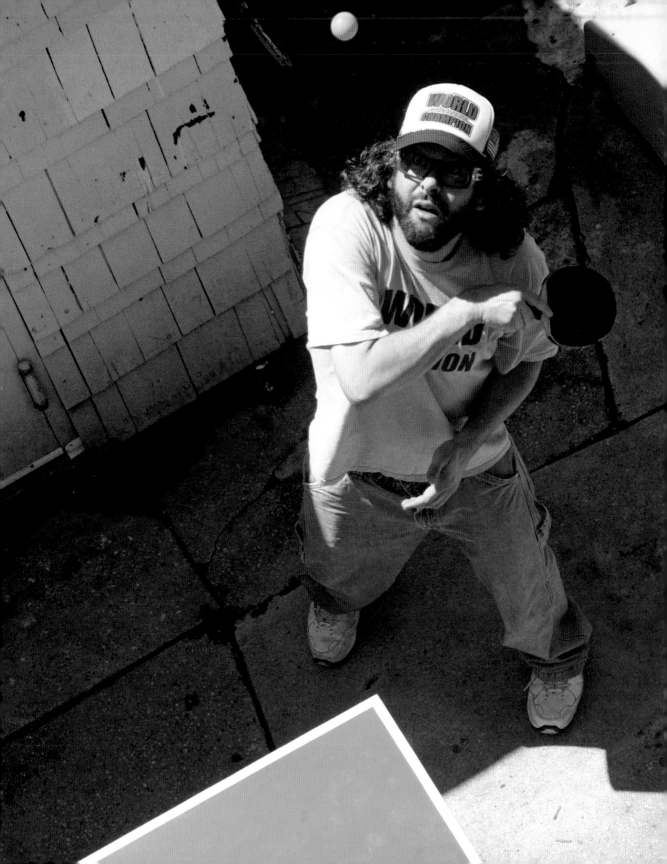

4

STARS: THEY'RE JUST LIKE US

PING PONG AND CELEBRITY

American society prides itself on being a meritocracy. And while one can argue our nation has no class system, only a fool would claim that the country is not segregated. The subtle pathways to power operate something like this: the beautiful people from every graduating high school class across the country are magnetically drawn to Los Angeles. New York sucks up the most ambitious and talented. The rest move to Chicago, apart from the puny brainiacs, once on the receiving end of daily school-yard beatings, who ultimately congregate as policy wonks in D.C. Crude stereotypes, perhaps, but true nonetheless. And the social cultures that they birth are as rigid as they are distinct. A good night out in Manhattan typically involves bottle service/

coke/having sex on piles of cash. Los Angelenos enjoy little more than dropping acid and searching for meaning while wandering around Runyon Canyon Park. And those in D.C. cower around a beer at the Hawk 'n ' Dove on Capitol Hill to discuss Sino-American grain policy and what the experience of touching a woman's breast might feel like.

It is rare that anyone or anything can break down these silos unless that person is Susan Sarandon and the thing is ping pong. In September 2009, Sarandon, long the thinking man's Samantha Fox, burnished her pedigree as the world's perfect woman by opening Spin, a luxurious ping pong club—nay, mecca—in downtown New York. The club was launched with appropriate hullabaloo at a *Vanity Fair*–sponsored party that anointed the forty-five square feet of the humble ping pong table as the singular place for Hollywood, Wall Street, and even the White House to collide amid the odor of cologne, worn rubber, and sweat. The ping pong zeitgeist was reinforced when the eclectic energy of the scene spawned a daring new magazine, *Celebrity Ping Pong,* with a vitality that made a mockery of the media industry collapsing all around it. *CPP* was the product of a brave visionary named James Cooper—advertising creative by day, the sport's Samuel Pepys by night.

But how did modest ping pong, a sport that has offered up so few celebrities of its own, quietly become as much a part of the celebrity pantheon as going to rehab for "exhaustion," reading *Dianetics: The Modern Science of Mental Health,* or being paid by Starbucks to publicly sip their beverages? Put another way, why do those successful strivers, with the world now at their feet, revert to the simple pleasures of pong? We consulted the sages, namely Corynne Steindler of the *New York Post*'s Page Six. Steindler opined, "Because it's easy to do between takes on a movie set or backstage at a concert. Plus, there's the added bonus of there being little chance of damaging one's face during the game." An expert answer, but one that did not fully satisfy us. If that was the only purpose, then why not the refuges of the pogo stick or the yo-yo? Mere subscribers to *Star* and *InTouch* magazine, we are hardly authorities on this subject, but if there is one thing we know about celebrities, it is that they are far from superficial individuals. And so we delved deeper into

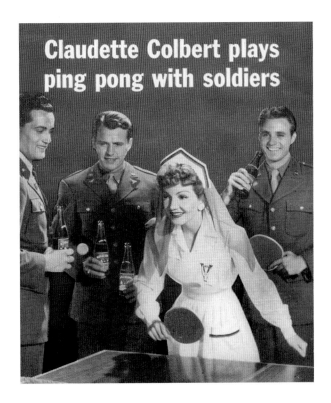

Claudette Colbert chooses Royal Crown Cola, circa 1943.

the relationship between Celebrity and Ping Pong, seeking to uncover the forces that have made it our century's Opus Dei.

1. Hollywood: The stars they shine so bright

In the dream factory that is Hollywood, everyone from DiCaprio (topless) and Sean Connery (topless) to Joan Crawford (fully clothed, but with more menace than the aforementioned duo combined) and Teri Hatcher relish ping pong. The list of enthusiasts in the movie industry reads like the cast of a Robert Altman flick. While we may think of ping pong bats in Hollywood being solely confined to seedy S&M dens, the vast majority are actually employed for their god-given purpose. The Incredible Hulk himself, Ed Norton, flies his coach around the globe to train on set. We remember the affair between Elizabeth Taylor and Richard Burton as one of frantic lovemaking followed by bouts of crockery smashing; in truth, the duo's relationship could not have been more

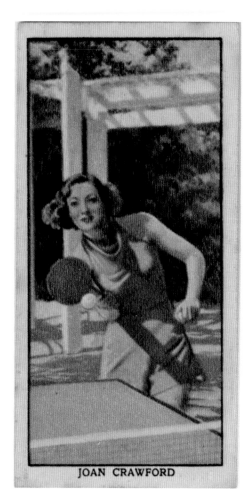

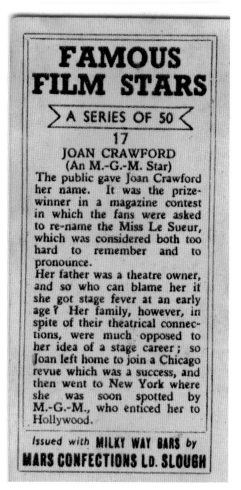

JOAN CRAWFORD

Joan Crawford demonstrates her unique grip of the paddle.

down-to-earth. They installed two ping pong tables in their home: one in the east wing to capture the morning light, the second in the west, so they could play and bask in the setting sun later in the day. Strip away the image and the hype, and *US* magazine is right: the stars are just like us. They never feel more human than when lulled by the rhythmic return of the ball across the net.

2. Wall Street: The table keeps your feet on the ground

The two men who graciously take turns as the richest being on earth, Warren Buffett and Bill Gates, know better than most that time is money. It is striking then that both reserve regular space on their schedules for bouts of ping pong. Indeed, in 2007 Buffett marked his seventy-fifth birthday by shipping the under-sixteen national champion, eleven-year-old Ariel Hsing, into his San Francisco celebrations. Hsing proceeded to trounce both the financier and his sideman, Gates. So tickled was Buffett that he repeated the performance before his shareholders at the annual Berkshire Hathaway meeting; Gates and he tag-teamed Hsing, this time unleashing simultaneous serves against her, yet they still fell to blissful defeat. Perhaps the two giddy titans were relieved to encounter a force more supreme than even their combined power: ubiquitous, omnipotent ping pong.

3. Uber-Athletes: Ping pong as a safety valve

Legendary athletes exist in a rare ether, blessed with superhuman ability reinforced by an intensity of focus. The same assets that make them without peer on the field of play often leave them bonkers amid the more mundane tasks of everyday living. Ping pong can provide a transition between the two worlds, an outlet for healthy competition away from the playing field. Bobby Fischer, the former World Chess Champion turned Icelandic anti-Semite, was a ping pong enthusiast. According to hardbat champion Marty Reisman, he approached the game the same way he played chess: "Fiercely, ferociously, going for his opponent's jugular. He was a killer, a remorseless, a conscienceless, ice-blooded castrator." No release there, then—and thus Fischer slowly went insane.

Back in the days when the world still considered the self-destructive sexaholic Tiger Woods to be a peerless golf-robot, the athlete found a more constructive role for his ping pong passion, using it to heal a professional rift with arch rival Phil Mickelson. Regular showdowns have offered a healthy release for Tiger, and a venue for Mickelson to triumph before the world's press: "You know, Tiger is an incredible athlete, in other areas, although he struggled with me at ping pong." Woods predictably turned the tables during their next showdown at the 2005 Ryder Cup in Virginia. Jack Nicklaus, then U.S. captain, reported that Tiger won, but Phil was handicapped by the fact

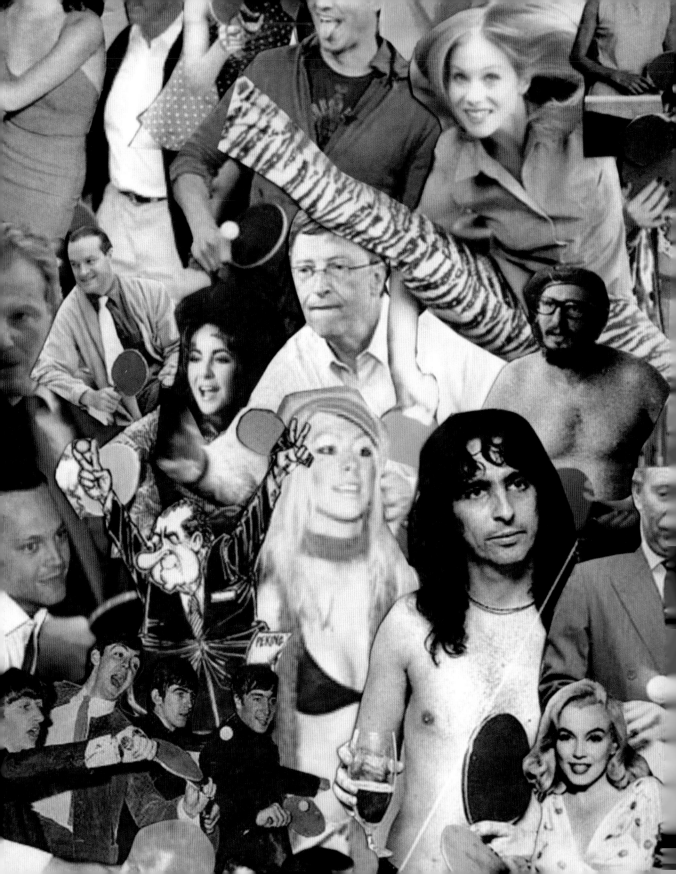

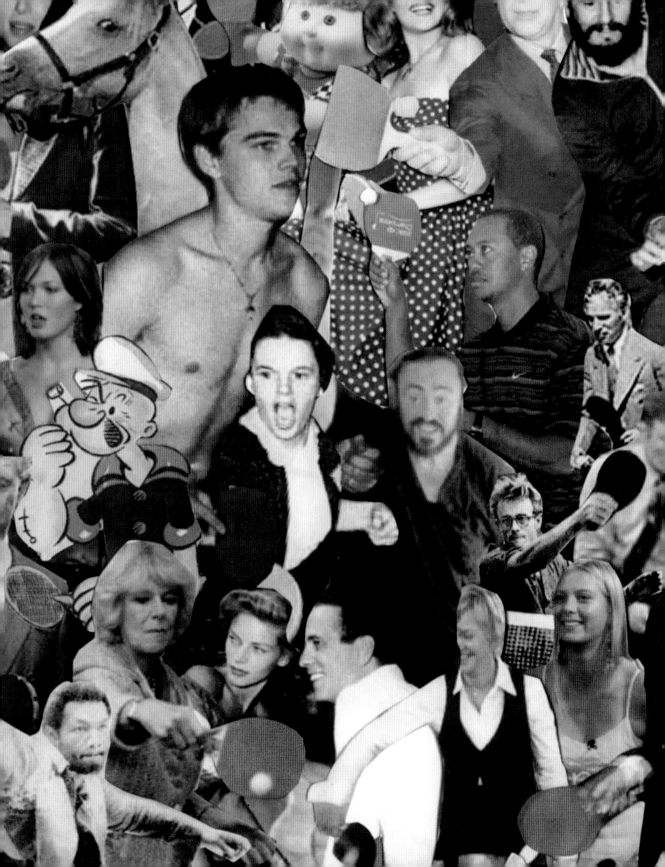

that a buffet counter was located too close to his behind, which cramped his natural form. As he had on the golf course so many times before, Tiger found a way to win by any means necessary. If only he had incorporated regular games of ping pong into his relationship with poor Elin, domestic bliss may have ensued.

4. Writers: The Game as Zen

Renowned journalist Harry Evans hosts a weekly ping pong parlor known as Print & Paddles, which has spawned a dizzying rivalry between A.J. Jacobs (the literary world's David Blaine) and mogul Mort Zuckerman (who is rumored to be a master of the unconventional art of rallying with bat in one hand and cell phone at the ready in the other). Salman Rushdie competes regularly at the home of surrealist painter Francesco Clemente. The Foer brothers hustle each other nightly in a Brooklyn basement. A ping pong paddle fits as smoothly into most writers' hands as a pen. But why? The founding bard of the obsession is Henry Miller, who battled Anaïs Nin at Clichy, Lawrence Durrell in Corfu, and Man Ray in Hollywood. Looking back on his bountiful life, Miller said, "This is my seventieth year of ping pong playing. I started at the age of ten on the dining room table. I take on players from all over the world. I play a steady Zen-like game. . . . No matter how glamorous an opponent may be I never let him, or her, distract me." Ping pong, in Miller's case, served as a mind-cleansing activity, powerful enough to blast through even the most challenging case of writer's block. (For more on Miller's pong exploits, see page 74.)

5. Music: PP as Rehab

The Beatles, ever the revolutionaries, compensated for their decidedly unorthodox grips by playing, predictably, as a foursome. Now 50 Cent hosts a "Naked Ping Pong Party" in Phoenix, Arizona, where half-stars such as Doug E. Fresh and Khloe Kardashian (inventor of the unique teeth whitening pen, Idol White) flashed their flair. Foo Fighter Dave Grohl takes a table on the road, cryptically revealing in an interview, "There's nothing wrong with a little

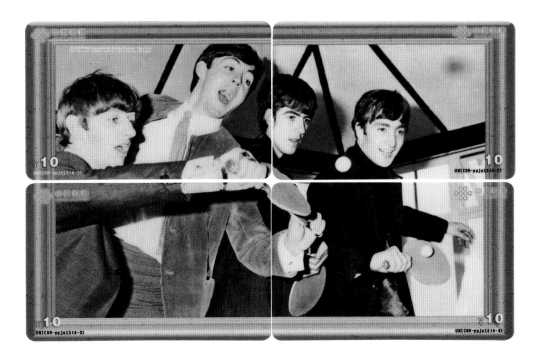

The Beatles with four paddles and two balls on set of four phone cards for Chinese Unicom phone company.

zhing-zhang now and again. We're big on it. There's no better way to warm up for a show than a nice five- or six-game tournament. It gets your hand-eye going; you break a sweat."

Sweating it out may be the key here. Primal Scream front man Bobby Gillespie shocked his fans by blaming his love of Colombian marching powder on his addiction to ping pong. "I used to do loads of cocaine. Me and my mates used to get sniffed up and play table tennis at my house. That's the way to do it. Put lines on the table and then you can do those Japanese topspins and backspins right. Cocaine and table tennis—it's a great recreational activity. That's when I'm at my best." Note to readers: if ever confronted by Gillespie, he is unbeatable in the first two games. Thus, challenge him to the best of five; hold on as best as you can at the outset and wait for fatigue to kick in and his skills to rapidly deteriorate.

The prolonged and frantic copulation between celebrity and ping pong has recently spawned two new minotaur-esque archetypes in the form of actor Judah Friedlander and athlete Biba Golic—a celebrity who is a ping pong master and, at long last, a ping pong player who has acquired the scent of celebrity. First, *30 Rock*'s scene-stealer Judah Friedlander, a peerless stand-up comedian whose act has long contained boasts of being the "World Champion of the World" at every sport, in addition to moonlighting as a Navy SEAL and Bigfoot expert. Hirsute and prone to exaggeration Friedlander may be—but his game is very real. During the 2008 Beijing Olympics, he found himself a man obsessed, staying up nightly until 5 A.M. to track the progress of the table tennis competition. The spectacle summoned a long-dormant passion from deep inside Friedlander—one that had first been forged in basements and rec centers across his hometown of Gaithersburg, Maryland. The game had once been such a part of his life that he had dedicated precious hours in the wood shop during eighth grade, painstakingly creating a miniature table just three feet long and crafting a bat out of particleboard. Watching his laptop, he knew it was time for his return.

Friedlander's return began at a local Korean club in Flushing, and he soon found himself addicted, barnstorming ping pong venues across New York both before and after sets at comedy clubs. Hitting the ball became the perfect panacea for the stress generated by the business side of the entertainment industry, and Frieldlander developed an unquenchable desire to master every surface. "I like to keep things as tricky as possible by experimenting with every rubber so I can play even with hardbat and sandpaper. I want to be able to pick up any surface and destroy everyone." Among celebrities he has no rival. "Every once in a while, people tell me about some actor who has skills but then I see them in person and they stink, although a guy who played a terrorist in the last season of that show *24* is reputed to be a good hardbat."

Friedlander sharpened his game at tournament after tournament, but once he started to become recognized, the game ceased serving as an escape. But rather than give it up, Friedlander realized ping pong needed promotion, and so he dedicated himself to that task. "The sport is full of such interesting

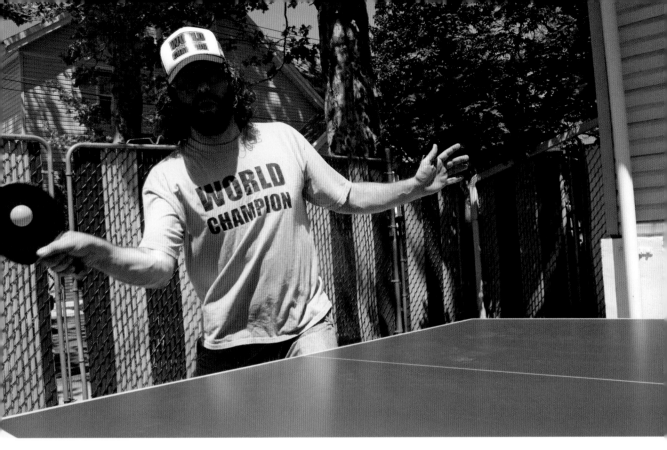

Judah Friedlander, world champion table tennis player extraordinaire, Queens, 2010.

people, and is so fucking fun and good for you, and yet the best players plow away in obscure clubs, playing for so little money—not unlike stand-up comedians. I wanted to lift ping pong above the radar." Friedlander has become a standard-bearer for the sport, hosting tournaments in Las Vegas and New York City and shooting a video for *Sports Illustrated* in which he destroys all comers, casually rallying through critical points whilst munching on a slice of pizza.

The ying to Friedlander's yang is Serbian-born ping pong pro Biljana "Biba" Golic—the blond beauty who has single-handedly attracted an army of awkward adolescent teens to the sport. Golic was dubbed the "Anna Kournikova of Table Tennis" by Robert Blackwell, the svengali of upstart equipment manufacturer Killerpsin, who plucked her from the hinterlands of Betzingen, where she toiled in obscurity on the German professional circuit. She began modestly

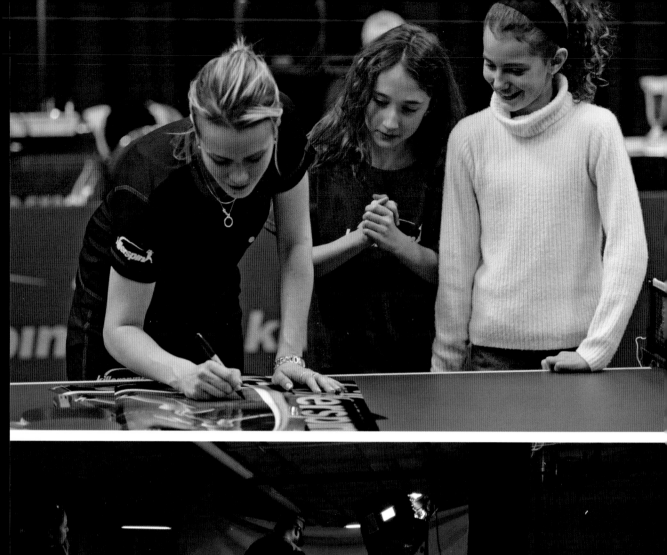
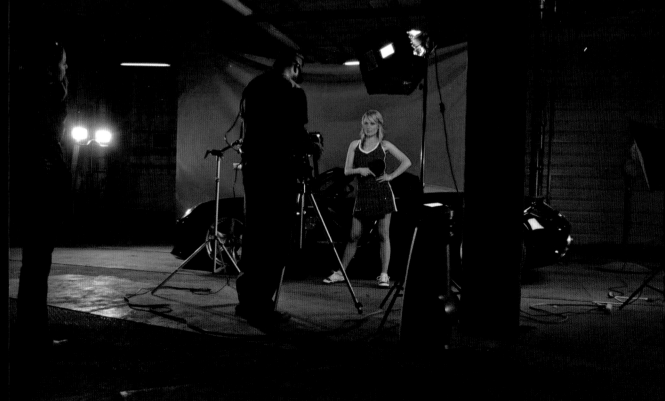

in the States, living in a Fort Worth Best Western on a table tennis scholarship at Texas Wesleyan, polishing both her game and her limited English skills. But once she joined the Killerspin ping pong tour, donned one of the brand's signature body-hugging red skirts, and began to thrash opponents both male and female, she instantly became the face of the brand. At only her second tournament, a grassroots fan base had developed. As Blackwell tells it, "There were over three hundred young guys sitting in the stands and these were not table tennis people. They were there for Biba." Fans bellowed her name in between points, a distraction Biba handled with good grace. One came equipped with a BIBA WILL YOU MARRY ME? sign—something even the great Victor Barna, a twenty-two-time world champion, never experienced in his pomp.

It did not take too long for the world's media to find her. She donned a pair of Daisy Dukes for a Rolling Stone "Hot List" photo shoot, ESPN summoned her to shoot a coveted promo ad, and then testosterone-soaked Spike TV crowned her its "Sexiest Sportswoman of the Year," an award for which she beat out Californian pole vaulter Allison Stokke. (The nominees were tastefully introduced with the tagline "One can work a pole, the other will paddle your ass; either way, losing has never been so sweet.") All of this exposure soon led to an avalanche of commercial opportunities. Biba was summoned to Vegas to play the real Anna Kournikova at table tennis. Then she was cast in the ping pong movie *Balls of Fury* and found herself strolling down the red carpet at a Hollywood premier. Like a snake eating its own tail, Biba is aware of the possible dangers of her sudden celebrity. The more famous she becomes, the less time she has to practice the game that thrust her into the spotlight in the first place, which is the unique differentiator setting her apart from the thousands of other blond red-carpet aspirants. "I have spent my whole life in table tennis. Playing it. Talking about it. Dreaming about it. There are a lot of pretty girls. I am a tennis player first of all, that is why I am here, and if I wasn't producing results no one would notice me." A wise woman's version of "between ping pong and celebrity, give me death."

Biba Golic, ping pong celebrity, role model, and billboard.

The Library of Champions

Celebrities are drawn toward ping pong like moths to a flame; that's been well documented, both here and elsewhere. Christian Bale picks up a paddle, shutters snap, and bloggers swoon: clockwork.

When a ping pong player seeks celebrity, however, it's a little trickier. The mainstream media sleeps on these champions. Fair and balanced? Until the names Samson Dubina and Ariel Hsing are popping from the cover of *US Weekly*, there's nothing fair about it.

Thus, world-class pongeurs soon learn to stop waiting for the paparazzi and instead take matters into their own hands. Historically, the first step on this path to stardom is to write (or at least "write") an instructional guide, a ping pong how-to. The content of these books is generally the usual mix of tips, strategies, and anecdotes, maybe with some overall life wisdom sprinkled throughout. But the real star-making moment comes on the cover. This must feature a vibrant photo of the player in action, generally midsmash. As with all action photos, the more action the better—extra points for ruffled hair, askew limbs, or at least a look of maniacal intensity. Throw in a flash of neon color, choose from a few awesome fonts, and print several hundred thousand copies. Fame and fortune is . . . possible. If the first volume doesn't have the desired effect, become better-looking and try again.

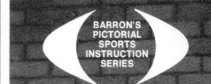

Chester Barnes: Table Tennis

BARRON'S
PICTORIAL
SPORTS
INSTRUCTION
SERIES

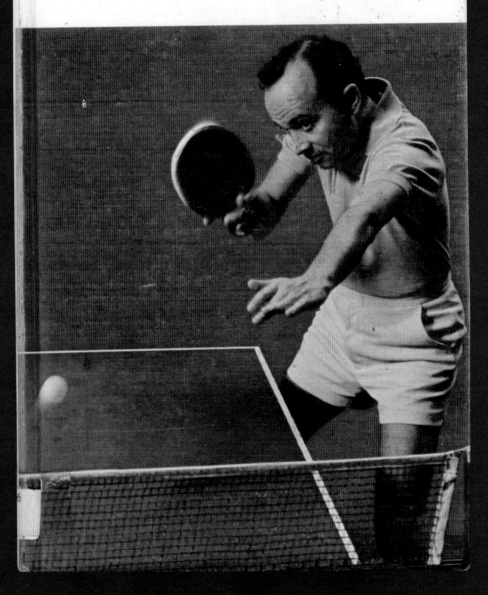

Sports Illustrated
Table Tennis

By Dick Miles

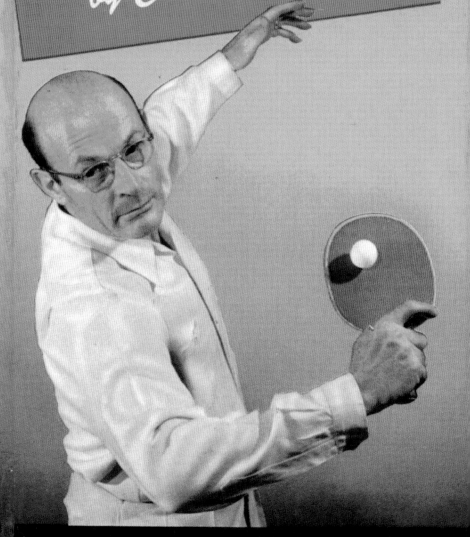

TABLE TENNIS
by Coleman Clark

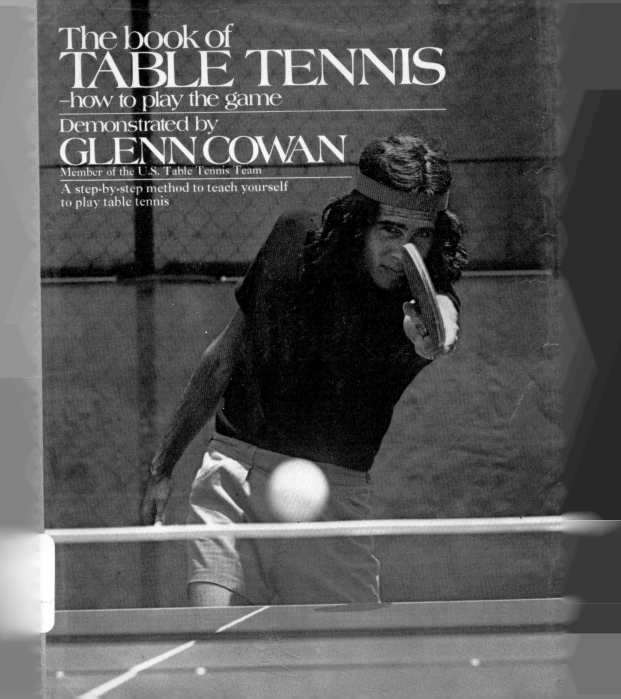

The book of
TABLE TENNIS
–how to play the game

Demonstrated by
GLENN COWAN

Member of the U.S. Table Tennis Team

A step-by-step method to teach yourself
to play table tennis

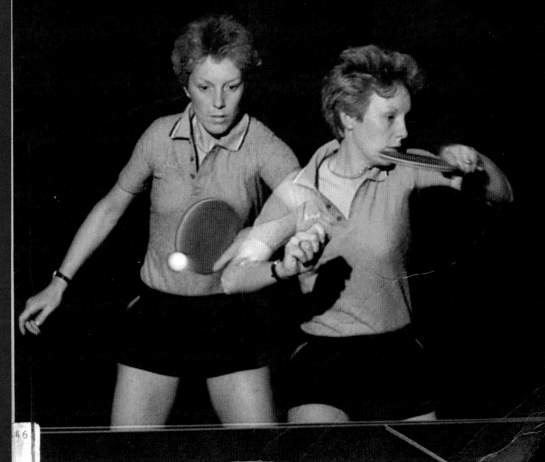

Top-class
Table Tennis
Jill Hammersley MBE
and Donald Parker

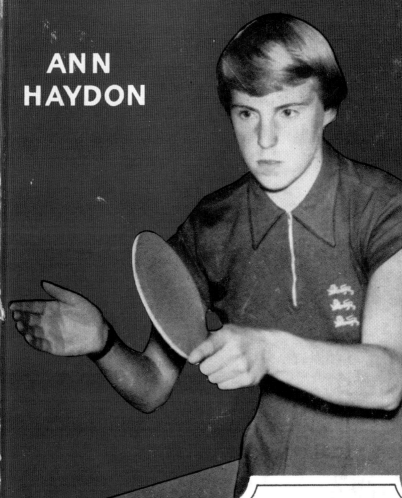

ANN
HAYDON

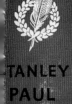

Tackle
TABLE
TENNIS
This Way

THE WAY TO THE TOP

Denis Neale

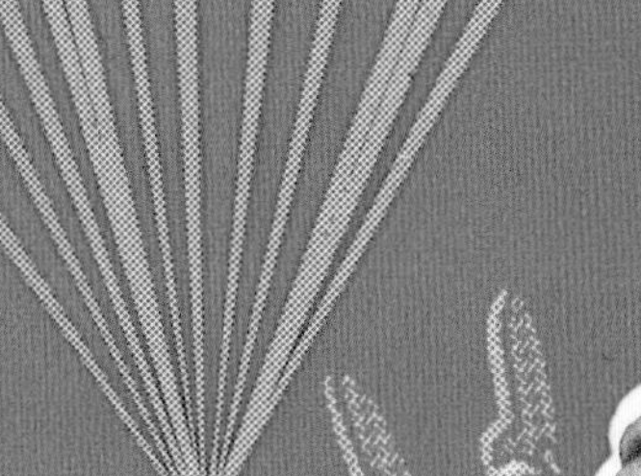

THE
WAY
TO
THE
TOP

Denis Neale

table tennis

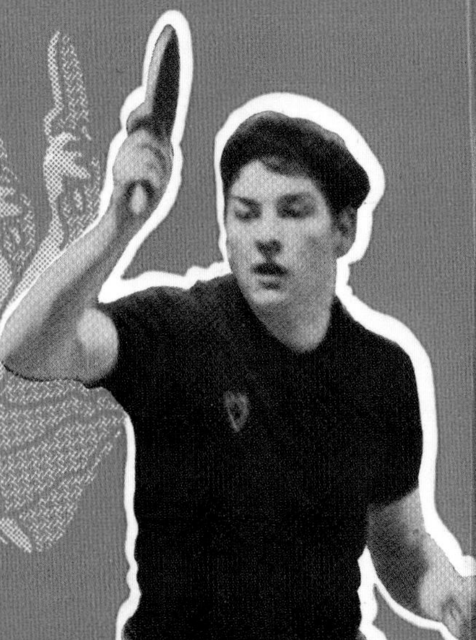

ARTHUR BARKER

table tennis

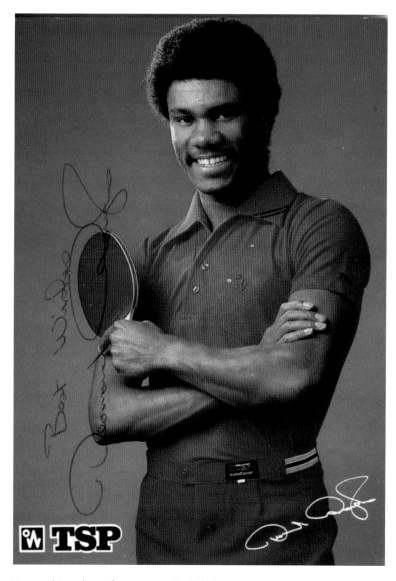

Desmond Douglas, a fourteen-time English champion, circa 1980.

NO PROPER SPORT
BY NICK HORNBY

I have no idea why I can remember the name of Desmond Douglas. I am at a loss to explain why, if someone asked me to come up with a table tennis player from the whole of world table tennis history, my list would begin and end with him. He was pretty good, clearly—British number one, European number three, world number seven—but these are rankings comparable with Tim Henman's, rather than Courier's, or Agassi's, or Federer's. (You will note the absence of a Briton in the second part of that analogy. There simply isn't one who could make it work. Virginia Wade? Remember her? No. I didn't think so.) In other words, he was better than most people, and, like, *miles* better than you and me.

But he wasn't the best. The only ping pong player I can name was, at his peak, seventh best. There is no other field of human endeavor, I suspect, in which I would only be able to name the seventh-best participant. (Writing could be an exception. Over here in the U.K., we have placed one of our own in the top slot; it's possible, though, that we are deluded by our own ignorance, and that six of those regrettably obscure Nobel Literature winners could kick his ass into the middle of next week. For all I know, Shakespeare's stats might be exactly the same as those of Desmond Douglas: British number one, European number three, world number seven.)

There is one plausible explanation for the familiarity, and it goes like this. We love our sport in the U.K. We love football the most; we also like cricket and rugby, although we are only really interested in those two when our international teams are involved. As we are not very good at anything, we can also become absurdly excited by Olympic athletes who look as if they might stand a chance of a medal. Many millions of us stayed up until three in the morning to watch our (field) hockey team beat the Germans to win gold in '88; star striker Sean Kerly came back a national hero, and I didn't have to look his name up on Wikipedia or anything, not even for the spelling. We haven't been too interested in hockey since. I wondered, briefly, whether Desmond Douglas belonged in the Sean Kerly category of famous British sportsmen, but I fear that his apparent lack of international success counted against him: however inept we are, we always manage to produce a national number one, in every single sport you can name.

But despite these occasional distractions, we always come back to football. Up until a decade or so ago, our football games were played exclusively on Saturday afternoons; as a consequence, that was when our two main TV channels broadcast two very long sports programs. The BBC had *Grandstand*, and the commercial channel offered *World of Sport*, and we watched them in our millions, not least because there was no daytime television during the week. The only real problem with these sports programs was that they had no proper sport to show.

At 12:30, two and a half hours before the games kicked off, there were half-hour preview shows; at 4:45, just as they were coming to an end, we watched a teleprinter chatter results out onto an on-screen piece of paper. But between 1:00 P.M. and 4:45 P.M. there was nothing.

They weren't allowed to show a match, on the grounds that we'd all stay home in front of the TV, instead of go to the stadiums; cricket is a summer game, and international rugby takes place only rarely. So those hours of broadcasting time—seven of them, over the two channels, in days when we only had three channels anyway—were filled with anything that could even loosely be described as sport. There was a lot of horse racing; there was show jumping, and the occasional athletics meet; there was swimming and badminton and squash and, yes, ping pong. And I suspect that this is how Desmond Douglas came to national prominence: he was young, and black—in the days when we didn't see too many black people on our TV screens—and for years he dominated a sport that provided crucial ballast for desperate broadcasters. Given that England's football team failed to qualify for the World Cup in 1974 and 1978, and didn't get very far in 1982 or '86, and it was only international football that the authorities allowed us to watch live, it is probable that Desmond Douglas was on our small screens more than our football idols.

Okay, I could have turned him off, but I clearly didn't. What else was there to watch? Now there are countless games of football televised every day of the week, games taking place in England, Scotland, Spain, France, Germany, Italy, anywhere, and I find those hard to turn off, too: to many generations of sports fans, the abundance seems like a miracle. Anyone who remembers Desmond Douglas spent a long time waiting—waiting for results, waiting for World Cups, waiting for the overhyped, overexposed, overanalyzed football world we have now.

Paul Drinkhall is Britain's current number one table tennis player apparently, but I couldn't tell you what he looks like. This may be because he's the world number 130, although I suspect that even if he were the best in the entire universe, we wouldn't be taking much notice, not when there's a live Wigan v. Blackburn game on TV. Sorry, Paul. But good luck anyway.

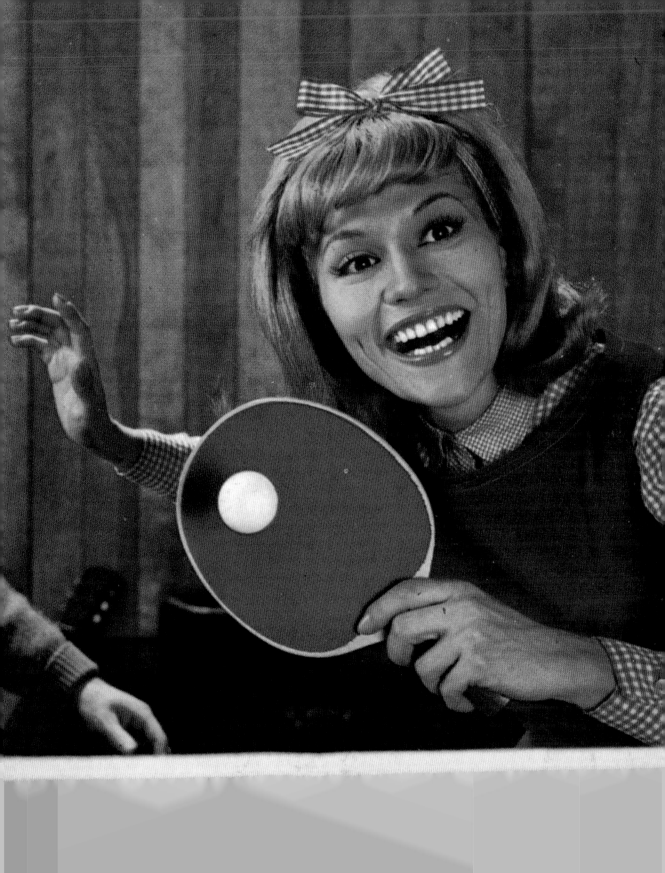

5

THE PADDLE OF YOUTH

AGING BODIES, DECAYING MINDS, AND THE QUEST FOR ETERNAL LIFE

In this game of kings, dwarves topple giants, chubsters crush bodybuilders, and wrinkled elders regularly whip whippersnappers. The same could be said for many pastimes—for example, chess or alcoholism. But ping pong is unique among these levelers; while it resists simple anatomical dominance, it is nevertheless intensely physical. Ping pong asks us to simultaneously inhabit our bodies and transcend them. We learn patience. We learn humility.

This helps explain ping pong's popularity as a lifelong pursuit. The race goes to the quick, but the match goes to the wise. Utterly egalitarian, ping pong has a home at every stage of our lives: the precocious child struggling to defeat an older brother; the power-mad stockbroker seeking instant adrenaline after the market closes; and most of all, the wily veteran, master of spins and master of minds. These silver foxes grow more devilishly dangerous with each passing year, seeking out youthful opponents and turning their spastic energy against them, judo-style. The game evolves with the player, revealing itself decade by decade. From humid Brooklyn clubs to humid Sarasota

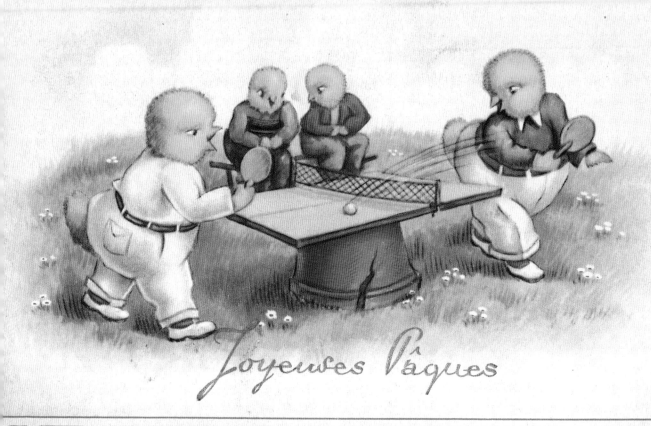

Joyeuses Pâques

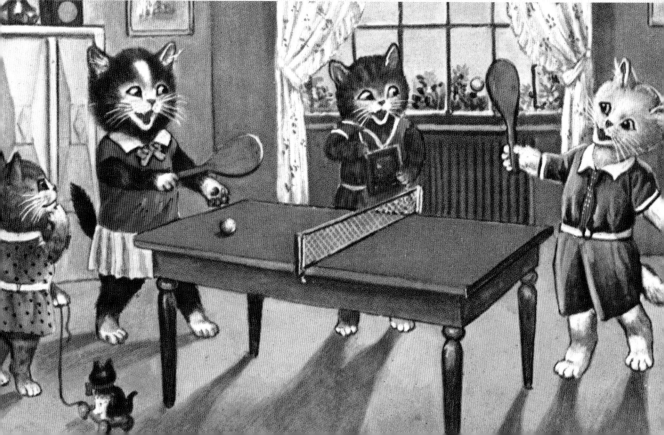

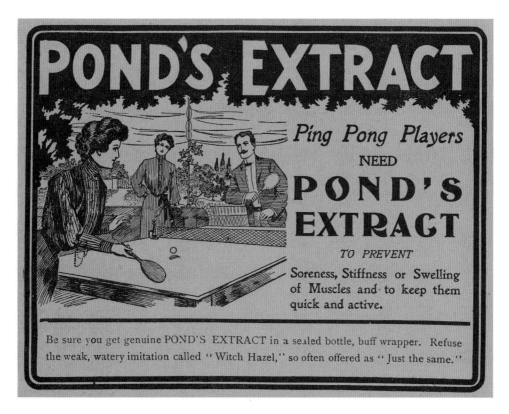

An early protection campaign against tenosynovitis from 1902. Note: Accept no imitations—witch hazel is not "just the same."

retirement communities, the ball bounces on and on, a game that never ages and keeps its devotees young.

Gerontologists recommend ping pong as a perfect activity for feisty oldsters: demanding yet sustainable, combines coordination and endurance, and calls upon multiple muscle groups, all with a low risk of injury. (This safety may be overestimated; as early as 1902, the *British Medical Journal* was reporting upon tenosynovitis, the dreaded "ping pong ankle." Thirty years later, the *New York Times* reported that "the sport is now considered more dangerous than bowls" and in 1944 recounted the story of Lieutenant Frances MacWilliams: "Flier hurt at ping-pong; had escaped without a scratch in fifty bombing missions.") Higher impact than shuffleboard, less soul-crushing than sidewalk strolls with crotchety neighbors—ping pong is a natural fit for golden-year exercise.

Left: Ping pong can be enjoyed by all ages and body types. Hundreds of these cards were illustrated in the early twentieth century, often focusing on cats but spanning the entire animal kingdom.

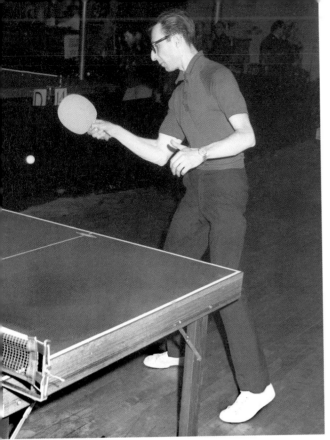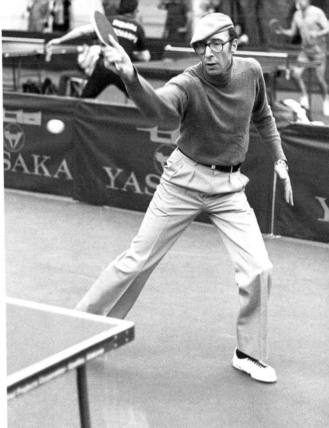

Marty Reisman, hardbat legend—unchanged through the years, preserved by ping pong.

But this is not just a hobby. The legendary Marty Reisman began at age twelve in a settlement house on the Lower East Side, won the U.S. Hardbat championship at age sixty-seven (the oldest person ever to win an open national competition in a racquet sport) and is still deadly as he enters his ninth decade. Dorothy De Low, born in *1912*, recently represented Australia in the World Veterans Games in Rio. Clearly this runs deeper than some nursing-home time waster. Is it possible that ping pong is actually *reversing* the effects of aging?

The aging process is not well understood by current medicine. Some cells die, others are born, and some are borderline immortal; some expire too fast, others last too long. Somehow this whole bundle of mush hangs around for forty million minutes, give or take a decade. What makes it go? What makes it stop? Why does the mayfly wilt after a single fluttery day, while Dorothy De Low is slamming her way through a new millennium?

A leading theory of organismal senescence is the Rate of Living Hypothesis. To oversimplify: live fast, die young. The slower you move, the longer you live. (The animal's size is also involved in the equation.) What animal has the longest life span? The giant tortoise, which has plodded through up to 177 years in captivity. The ol' tortoise does not hurry through these years. In fact, most animals have approximately the same number of heartbeats over the course of a life—somewhere in the ballpark of 2,500,000,000 thumps.

So here's one possible way to extend your life: sit very still. Don't get too excited. Don't waste any heartbeats. Also, no dessert; recent experiments have significantly extended the life span of lab mice by severely restricting their caloric intake, thereby slowing metabolism. Scientists aren't yet sure whether this also applies to humans, but it might—give it a try. A quiet, hungry, boring life might earn you a few extra years tacked on to the end.

Or you could try the Way of the Bat. The bat? The bat. The Rate of Living Hypothesis holds true as a general rule, but there are exceptions—most notably, our spooky winged friends. Approximately mouse size, bats would be expected to hang around for three or four years. But they live longer than that—a lot longer. Ten times as long, in fact; bats born during the Carter administration are just now heading for the Great Cave in the Sky.

As a result, bat aging is a hot topic among gerontologists trying to unlock the secrets of long life. Maybe someday we'll be able to isolate the vital chromosome or enhanced protein homeostasis or whatever, but until then our best bet may be to just emulate the bat lifestyle. Not all of it, of course—no one is suggesting that we sleep upside down or eat only bugs. But the *essence* of chiropteran life is not far from our grasp. Constant readiness. Quick, darting motions. Intercepting small objects in their path of flight. No hiding in mouse holes, no nibbling bits of scavenged cheese, but rather action, reaction, swoops, strikes. Sound familiar? Could it be? It could: our old friend ping pong, perhaps the most batlike of human endeavors.

Ping pong even demands that quintessential bat skill: echolocation. Bats

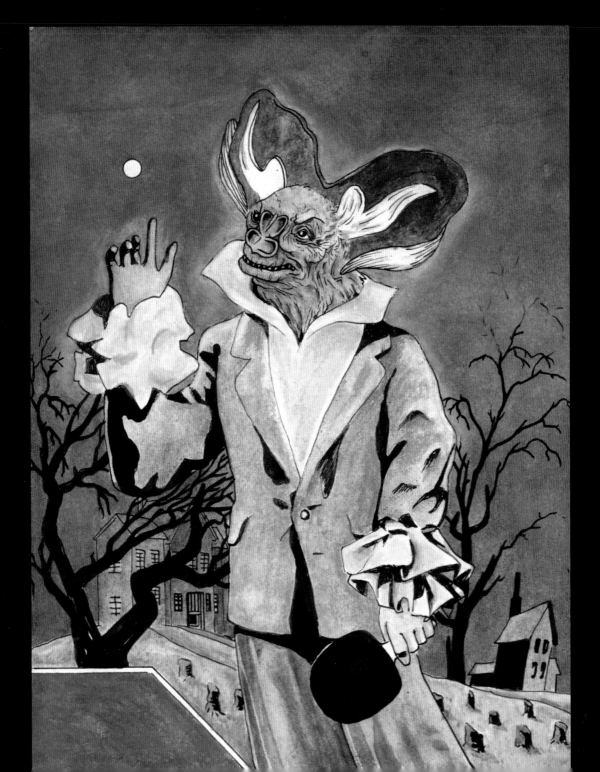

famously find their prey not by sight but by sound—bouncing high-pitched chirps off buggy bodies in the night. In ping pong, the ball moves too fast to catch with sight alone; sonic data, the musical ping and pong, are also vital. Describing the infamous switch from hard pongy paddles to silent sponges, Marty Reisman has lamented, "It was as if I were deprived of one of my senses. You're conditioned to react to the plickety plock, and this sponge caused dead silence."[1]

For the ultimate testament to the level of precision possible in ping pong echolocation, consider the case of Charles M. "Chuck" Mednick, one of the top ping pong referees of the 1950s. Mednick set a record by scoring fifty-four matches in one day at the 1953 National Table Tennis Championships. Mednick was also blind—blind as a bat, you might say. Said Mednick: "I just do something a blind man can do well—make his ears and sense of location work for him."

The conclusion is unexpected, but the logic is clear: bats live far beyond the simple dictates of the animal kingdom, and ping pong is the most batlike of all human endeavors. We cannot be *certain* that a strict regimen of therapeutic ping pong will lead us all past the century mark, but it sure beats the other options (calorie restriction, omega–3 enemas, etc).

Of course, physical decay is only half the problem. What of the persistent Alzheimic nightmare? What good is a supple ponging bod if the mind slips into hazy dementia? Chiroptera, unfortunately, does not provide guidance here; the scientific literature shows no studies on elderly bats attempting to solve bat crosswords. What can we do to keep our minds in serve-ready alertness?

Almost 10,000 brain cells die every day, pong or no pong—and once those cells are gone, they're probably gone for good. (The decay rate varies, of course; if you happen to be fond of the scent of paint thinner, you can burn through 300,000 cells in one glorious, dreamy day.) Previously it was thought that once a cell dies, a pathway breaks, and soon you can't remember where you parked the car; this is known as the Neuronal Fallout model. This model, however,

---

1. We won't even mention that the proper term for a ping pong paddle is actually *bat*. This is a serious investigation, not some mash of easy puns.

The immortal vampiric pongeur, depicted by artist Niklas Nenzén.

has been contradicted by recent evidence showing that the brain is more flexible than previously believed; the brain interacts with its environment, constantly evolving and adapting throughout life.

One implication of this Brain Plasticity model is that what you do affects how you think; the brain can be exercised like a muscle. Activities that require fast, accurate mental processing help develop new neural pathways and stimulate the neuromodulatory machinery. Ping pong isn't the *only* activity that fits these criteria, but . . . well, don't just trust me; Dr. Daniel Amen, author of *Making a Good Brain Great,* makes it official: "Table tennis is the world's best brain sport."

To skeptics, this might all still sound a bit *circumstantial.* "Bats? Plastic brains? Hrmph! Show me the proof. Show me an experiment *specifically* examining the effect of ping pong on brain activity." Well, okay, since you asked: please refer to Teruaki Mori and Tomohiko Sato's study in volume 17 of the Japanese biomechanics journal *Baiomekanizumu.* The results were, I mean, wow. First, take a look at those graphs or whatever—very impressive. Second, photon tomography showed increased brain blood flow after pong play—nice. Third, a group of 2,900 players were shown to have a lower level of "dotage" than a similar group of nonplayers (what a sad double whammy for that control group—first an empty, colorless life, and then senility at the end). Finally, brain-disease patients with a ping-pong-based rehabilitation program displayed decreased dementia and depression.

What should we make of these groundbreaking results? A fluke? Biased, pong-crazy researchers? *Is it possible that ping pong actually keeps our brains strong?*

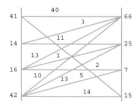 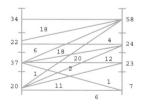 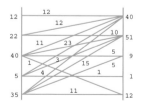

Mori and Sato's groundbreaking *Baiomekanizumu* data.

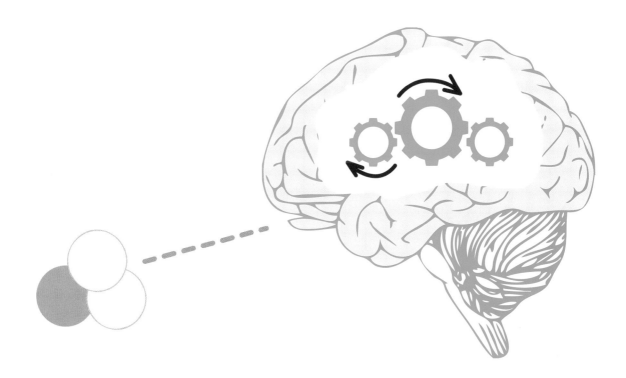

We are approaching fairly stupendous territory here, so let's review: there is both anecdotal (De Low, Reisman, etc.) and physical (gerontological studies, bat breakthroughs, etc.) evidence indicating that ping pong may be an ideal activity to counter the effects of aging. There is a theoretical framework explaining why ping pong may provide a batlike exception to standard life span limits. There is increasing evidence that ponglike exercises may directly circumvent the neural effects of senescence. There is *specific data* showing that ping pong improves mental activity and decreases brain disorders.

The strands of unexpected connections are beginning to weave together into something larger—a web of possibility, a lattice of support, a scaffold of palatial proportions . . . or, dare we say it, a fountain of youth. Is it possible that poor Ponce was just a few centuries too early? Were that dreamy Spaniard to land in Florida today, he still wouldn't find the bubbling brook of his dreams— but he might encounter John Donnelly of Sun City Center, recent table tennis gold medalist at the National Senior Games. Donnelly is 103.

Clearly, ping pong has much to teach medicine, and medicine is listening. But it would be folly to think this conversation goes in only one direction. Ping pong may allow us to play long into the future, but what kind of future will this be? More importantly, what kind of ping pong will we play? Most precisely, what kind of *we* will be playing that future pong?

Big questions like this require big thinkers, brains unconfined by arbitrary details of the moment. We're now edging into the realm of transhumanism—the speculabiotechnollectual movement exploring how technological advances can enhance our basic human capacities and perhaps eliminate aging entirely. These goals have relevance beyond ping pong—e.g., foosball—but you can see how transhumanism would hold special attraction for a pongeur entering the golden years. The movement is full of speculative rhetoric along the lines of:

> Posthumans could be completely synthetic artificial intelligences, or they could be enhanced uploads, or they could be the result of making many smaller but cumulatively profound augmentations to a biological human. The latter alternative would probably require either the redesign of the human organism using advanced nanotechnology or its radical enhancement using some combination of technologies such as genetic engineering, psychopharmacology, anti-aging therapies, neural interfaces, advanced information.
> (Nick Bostrom, of Humanity+, a leading transhumanist organization)

But they also laughed at Edison, know what I mean? Or maybe they didn't laugh, but they certainly would have poked fun at him on the blogosphere—and skeptics didn't invent the phonograph. Sometimes a bit of grandiose speculation is necessary to let us see beyond our own noses. And this speculation is not only the realm of free-thinking techno-hippies. The good ol' Department of Defense has commissioned studies on possible military uses of "Human Performance Modification"—the brain-computer interface (i.e., neural implants, possibly paired with prosthetic weapons), plasticity-enhancing neuromodulators, etc.—and concluded, basically, yes.

In fact, we don't even need to look far beyond our aforementioned noses to see the early transhumanist indicators that are already upon us. Athletics

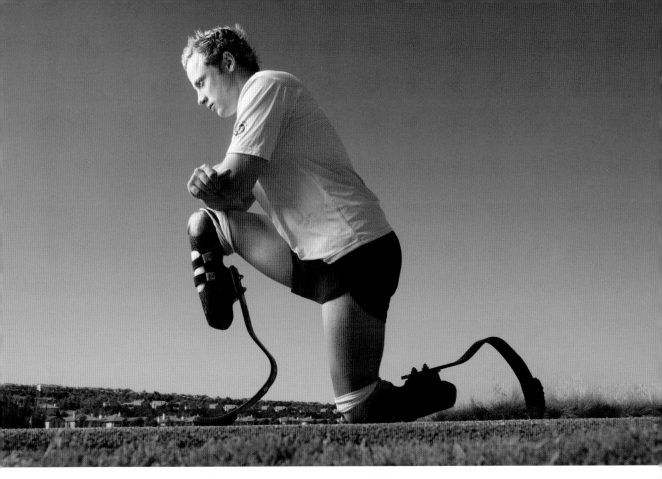

Oscar Pistorius, a South African quarter-miler and possible 2012 Olympian.

has always been a fertile ground for human enhancement technology (HET), and so the 2008 Beijing Olympics serve as a useful capsule of current efforts to transcend our anatomical limitations.

The months before these Olympics provided perhaps the most vivid appearance of HET on a public stage: Oscar Pistorius, a young South African who had both legs amputated as an infant. Now wearing Össur Flex-Foot Cheetah prosthetics, Pistorius has become a world-class quarter-miler. Nicknamed "Blade Runner" for his distinctively shaped "legs," many argued that Pistorius's replacements gave him an unfair advantage over the original. Pistorius ultimately fell seven-tenths of a second short of the Olympic qualifying time in the 400 meter, but he is determined to try again for the 2012 Games in

Next page: Topio, Vietnamese table tennis player, possible 2024 Olympian.

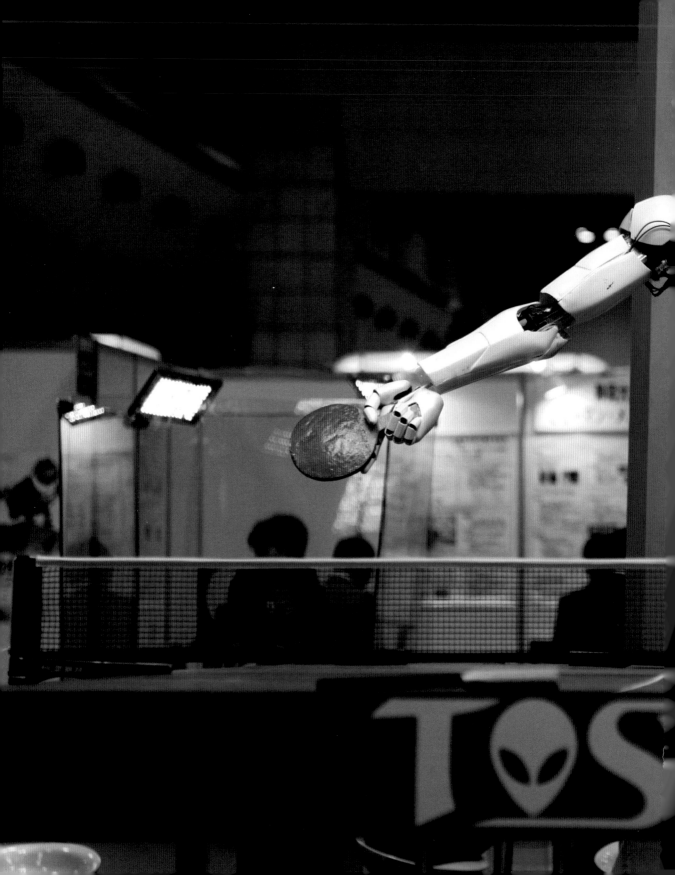

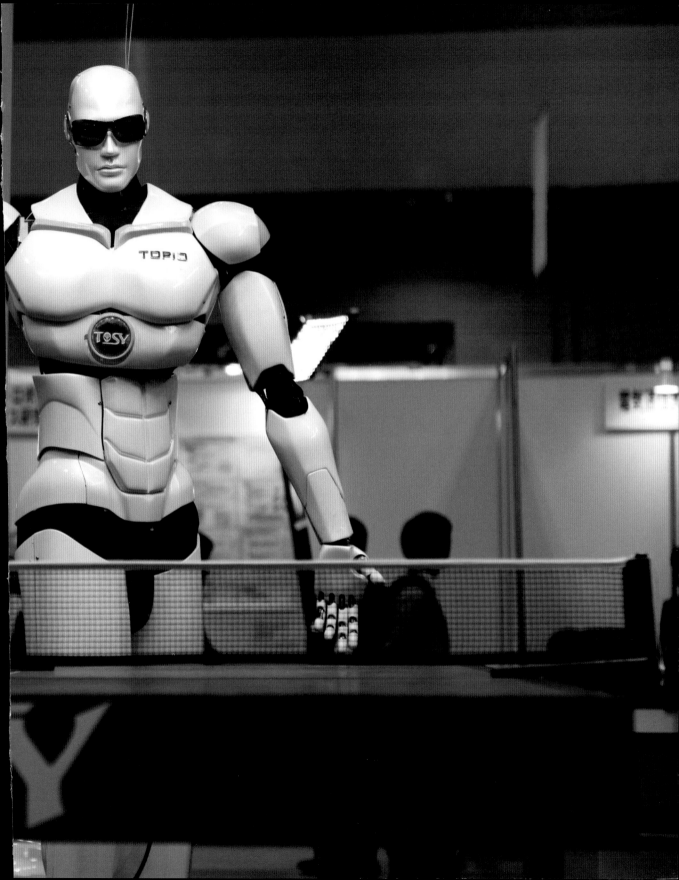

London; whether the eventual trailblazer is him or some yet-unknown young amputee, the scenario is already far more than mere speculation.

Even with these more futuristic developments temporarily out of sight, human enhancement pervaded these Olympics nevertheless, via a more traditional form of biotechnological fiddling: drugs. Testing for performance-enhancing substances at the Beijing Olympics saw athletes disqualified across the full spectrum of events—not just traditional cocktail sports like wrestling and cycling, but also seemingly innocent competitions like fencing, canoeing, pistol shooting, and show jumping. Show jumping! Equine enhancement technology! The point is, the transhumanist future—intentional amputation, downloaded brains, robotic butlers, a dream for some and a nightmare for others—is in fact a transhumanist *present*.

Which brings us to the question: where is ping pong in all this? As we've observed elsewhere, ping pong is usually at the forefront of any fundamental shift in the human experience, be it technological, political, or romantic. And this transhumanist evolution seems like it would be no exception. Just think of it: the *Beijing* Olympics, prosthetics and chemicals abounding, China plowing millions of dollars into its quest to sit atop the medal count . . . and here comes the national sport, the standard-bearer of a people (see Chapter 6). The hunger for absolute dominance must have been tremendous.

And so where was China's bionic pong warrior? A six-million-dollar man, with a bit of RoboCop if they were feeling ambitious? Or at least an Ivan Drago type, injected to the gills, muttering "I will break you" at trembling opponents across the net?

None of these appeared. Instead, China made do with actual nonmedicated, nonmetallic human beings. Why did China settle for these outdated contraptions of flesh and bone? Why didn't they make something better?

Because they couldn't. When it comes to humble, persistent ping pong, the focused might of the largest nation on Earth could not improve upon the original human machine. In almost every other sport, enhancements and refurbishings abound; entire agencies and laboratories have been constructed specifically to prevent athletics from picking this ripe fruit. Ping

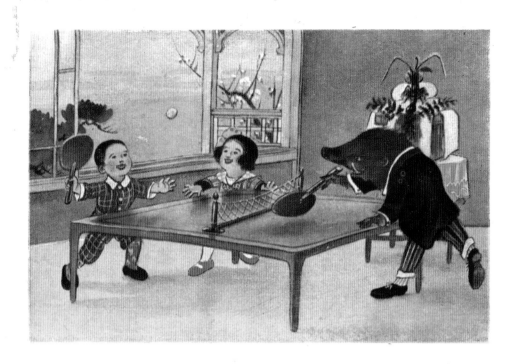

Despite technological advancements, humans still cannot be defeated by robots, nor by wild boars.

pong, however, provides its own prevention; the unique, delicate balance of mind and body, of precision and power, of competition and craftiness resisted any attempt at enhancement. In the centuries to come, who knows; perhaps scientists deep in the Mongolian steppes are already developing a being of pure elastic energy, with spongy paddles sprouting directly from wrists and neck. But for the moment, our homely, pre-post-human frame may in fact be the ideal ping pong creation. And is this not strangely inspiring? Isn't there a certain pride in this? When we pick up that paddle, we are, in a way, being most truly *ourselves*. Playing ping pong does not just keep us young; it may, in fact, keep us human.

Health Hazards

Do you remember the days when we still believed cigarettes were good for us? When a pack of Joes appeared to offer friends, fun, and the spirit of individuality instead of lung cancer, heart disease, and emphysema? In those happy days of the 1950s, adult Americans puffed on a staggering 2,558 cigarettes per capita a year. *Everyone* was inhaling, as an ad for Camel helpfully illustrated: "Three nationally known independent research organizations asked 112,597 doctors to name the cigarette they smoked. More doctors named Camel than any other brand."

How did Big Tobacco lure the country into lighting up? By co-opting the purity of the ping pong lifestyle and perverting it in the name of Marlboro Country. Exhibit A would be the 1947 ad in which Mary Reilly, the American table tennis sensation, reaches perkily for a selection of forehands, before breaking for a Camel, proclaiming, "Experience is the best teacher . . . in playing table tennis or choosing a cigarette."

Thanks in part to Ms. Reilly, Camel became the leading brand, pumping out over ninety-eight billion smokes a year, and soon everyone else was getting in on the ping pong action. Glowing in their matching neckerchiefs, a doubles combo enjoy the relaxing effect of a shared Pall Mall, in sharp contrast to their nonsmoking opponents, who remain drenched in sweat. A barely sober Spud smoker, lecherous in a tuxedo, leans against the table, rally interruptus. And a Kool-smoking suburban couple, Harold and Alice Burns, advocate weekend smoking, suggesting the world enjoy the mild menthol of their favorite brand to "smooth your throat" and "clear your mind of every thought of bosses and time clocks."

There is a dimension of fantasy in the retrospectively quaint yet utterly manipulative combination of ping pong and tobacco. The Camel ad introduces us to the pseudo-science of the "T-Zone"—the "proving ground for any cigarette." *T* stood for both *taste* and *throat,* which presumably was shorthand for "tastes terrible" and "throat cancer." But some have resisted the reality that smoking causes one in five deaths that occur in the States annually. Matthew Syed, a former English table tennis number one turned journalist, noted that the Greek ping pong team would light up in between games throughout the 2008 Olympics. In the world of ping pong, old habits die hard.

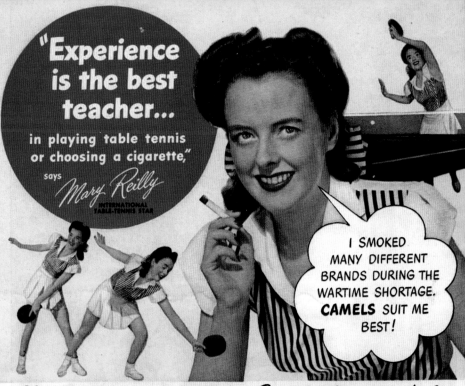

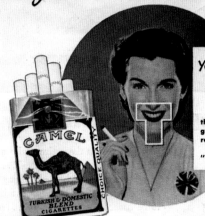

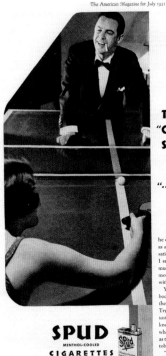
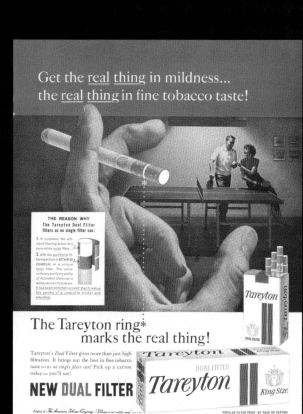

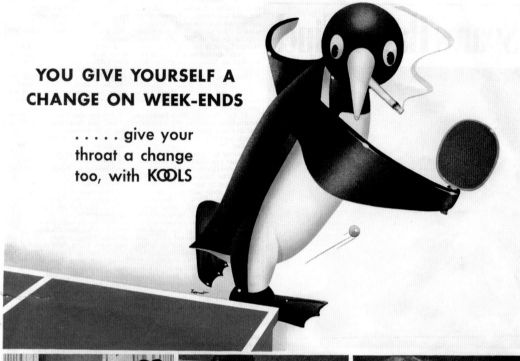

YOU GIVE YOURSELF A CHANGE ON WEEK-ENDS

. . . . . give your throat a change too, with **KODLS**

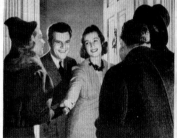

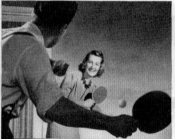

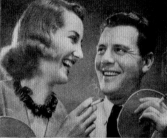

FRIDAY'S THE NIGHT when Harold Burns likes company to call . . . and Alice does, too. You see, Harold works like a beaver all week long, but when the *week-end* arrives, he likes to *forget* work . . .   and take it real easy.

ENJOY YOURSELF, GANG! Just clear your mind of every thought of bosses and time clocks. Say! I see you leave week-day things *completely* behind by switching from your regular cigarettes to **KODLS** over the week-end! Good going!

THAT TOUCH of mild menthol feels so soothing to the throat, *every* smoker should try this week-end plan. Do it now! You'll soon want **KODLS** for your *steady* smoke! And save the coupons, good in the U. S. A. for *premiums*.

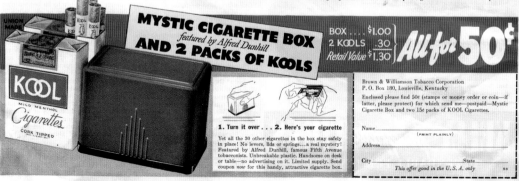

MYSTIC CIGARETTE BOX
featured by Alfred Dunhill
AND 2 PACKS OF KOOLS

BOX	$1.00
2 KOOLS	.30
Retail Value	$1.30

All for 50¢

KOOL
MILD MENTHOL
Cigarettes
CORK TIPPED
UNION MADE

1. Turn it over . . . 2. Here's your cigarette

Yet all the 30 other cigarettes in the box stay safely in place! No levers, lids or springs...a real mystery! Featured by Alfred Dunhill, famous Fifth Avenue tobacconists. Unbreakable plastic. Handsome on desk or table—no advertising on it. Limited supply. Send coupon *now* for this handy, attractive cigarette box.

Brown & Williamson Tobacco Corporation
P. O. Box 180, Louisville, Kentucky
Enclosed please find 50¢ (stamps or money order or coin—if latter, please protect) for which send me—postpaid—Mystic Cigarette Box and two 15¢ packs of KOOL Cigarettes.

Name
(PRINT PLAINLY)
Address
City   State
This offer good in the U. S. A. only   55

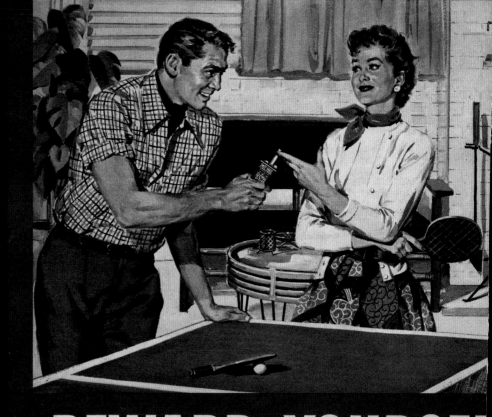

REWARD YOURSEl

Refresh yourself with "freshly-lit" flavor

In today's high-speed living, the smooth, gentle mildness of a freshly-lit PALL MALL encourages you to ease up . . . put worries aside . . . enjoy life more. Reward yourself with frequent moments of relaxation — get that certain feeling of contentment. Choose well — smoke PALL MALL.

Tastes "freshly-lit" puff after puff

PALL MALL is so fresh and fragrant, so mild and cool and sweet it tastes freshly-lit puff after puff.
Get pleasure-packed PALL MALL in the distinguished red package today.

Fin

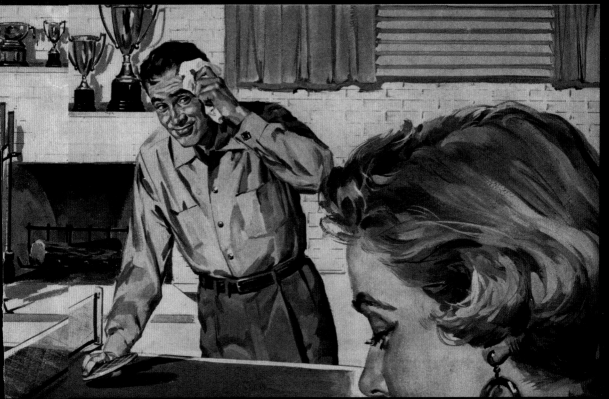

Your appreciation of PALL MALL quality has made it America's most successful and most imitated cigarette.

F... with the pleasure of smooth smoking

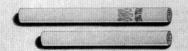
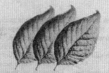
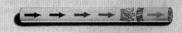

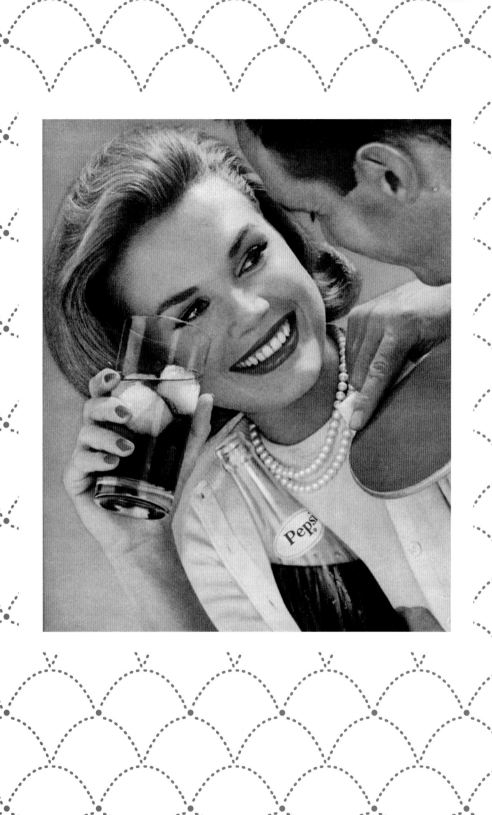

THE LIFE PURSUIT

BY HOWARD JACOBSON

I have never met an ex–table tennis player. Once you've played table tennis you go on playing no matter how old you are or how long it's been since you competed seriously.

This needn't mean that you actually wield your bat or climb back into your shorts, though veteran table tennis is going strong throughout the world and there are many players who go on competing into their eighties and beyond—strapped up, patched and bandaged, but still fighting for every point. Nor do I mean retrospectively, though retrospection is intrinsic to the game—the narrow margins you lost by, the humiliations you suffered, the chances you squandered, staying with you all your life. Of course you remember the victories too, though victory counts for less in table tennis than in most other sports, and you will remember the times you lost more often than you remember the times you won, even if that means bending the truth to your disadvantage. Only recently, at an entirely unassociated event, I met a person I hadn't seen for more than forty years who remembered losing to me 22–20 in the final game of a three-set match that decided the winner between Oxford and Cambridge. I too remembered the match and the score, only I recalled losing to him. We are still arguing over it by e-mail, each of us continuing to claim a famous defeat.

But this is not what I have in mind when I talk of the game staying with you. I mean philosophically. Table tennis, once you have played it with any purpose, becomes the very model for experience itself. In its quick-fire, ironic music—the ball coming back at you faster than thought—you hear the rhythms of reflective conversation and the best exchanges of wit when minds are alert. Table tennis lowers expectation and teaches you to live with disappointment as a necessary function of human engagement. But from the shapeliness of the game, its amused defeatism and quiet undemonstrativeness, you draw consolation, too. When I played it as a boy it seemed to make a little room an everywhere; now as man I see that it made an everywhere a little room.

In hours of sleeplessness I go through games I played decades before, trying to win matches I lost, hoping that with the experience of age I can now outwit those to whom I suffered a crushing or an unjust defeat. So far I have not yet played a single point any better than I did at the time, or overturned a single decision. Where I was beaten I go on being beaten. Where the net intervened in my opponent's favor, it still intervenes in my opponent's favor; where my down-the-line forehands just failed to clip the table, they go on missing by the same fraction.

It is an interesting question why I don't remember the games I won. But then where would be the point of replaying those? Best to leave well alone. I don't want suddenly to be losing to people I thrashed.

It is a masochistic sport. Perhaps not for the Chinese, who these days rarely taste defeat and who play at a far more frenetic pace than the great American and European players ever did. But for even the greatest European and American players of today, who labor to keep up with the Chinese, the game is more about loss than success. And for those who play at a more modest level, loss is of the essence. This is not to devalue table tennis; on the contrary it is to point out its superiority to all other sports where the neuroticism of having to win and remain in peak condition is paramount.

When Federer lost to Nadal in the final of the Australian Open Tennis Championships in 2009, he wept like a baby. Not only because he'd lost this match, but because he realized his impregnability was over. I cannot say for certain that no table tennis player in a similar position would do the same, but it is against the spirit of the game. Of course one loses. Of course the illusion of one's impregnability is gone forever. Table tennis is an unillusioned game. We choose the game—I don't say consciously—because we accept that defeat is inevitable, and we play to reconcile ourselves to its bitterness. You could say that we play because we know we have lost at something else already.

In this it is like art. The well-regulated rarely take up art. Why would you bother to remake the world if it were already fine in your eyes? Those who have no ambition to live in a different sort of world go on to play football or to enter banking. These are the conditions of life; you accept them and within their terms attempt to make a go of things. The artist feels otherwise: he is ill at ease in the world and must make it differently. If history is written by the winners, art is made by the losers. I don't mean that derogatively. You can be a loser and still triumph. But the sphere in which you triumph is not truly valued by the mass of mankind for whom success in the world is what counts.

Table tennis is to sport what art is to finance or politics. There have been great sportsmen and women who have succeeded at table tennis and lawn tennis—lawn tennis being a quintessentially conventional pastime. Fred Perry prospered in both. Ann Jones the same. But they are rare. Normally the temperament necessary for the one makes the other unattractive and unavailable to you. Lawn tennis, or tennis proper, as people who don't get ping pong call it, is in all its essentials an extrovert sport. You play in the daylight. The strokes you play are expansive. You raise the racket above your head. You leap for balls. You cover distances, you dash, you dive, you fall. Your body is on display. Not for nothing are many tennis players noisy breathers, exclaimers, and ejaculators. In tennis, nothing remains within your body, private to you. You don't hide your feelings. You are on display. You punch the air. You weep. You are the property of the crowd. And with that understanding crowds come to watch you. In every sense lawn tennis is public and you must be something of a publicity seeker to play it well.

Table tennis could not be more different. The shy are attracted to the game the moment they see it being played. No one is watching—so you do not have to fear exposure. The table and the playing area are confined, and to that degree you know from the start the limits of what will be expected of you. You can play close to yourself, the bat never an extravagant extension of you as a tennis racket is, your arm moving in immediate response to a private thought. Although you are closer to your opponent than you are in tennis, the introversion of the playing conditions reduces intimacy. Opponents rarely eyeball one another in the course of a game of ping pong. You look only into yourself, at your bat when it lets you down, at the table when the other person does something remarkable. It is not uncommon to wipe the table, though there is nothing on it, like Lady Macbeth vainly trying to wash away the memory of evil. In table tennis you do not shout at yourself as other sportsmen do, nor would you think of querying the decision of the umpire; you remonstrate, if you must, quietly, as befits the cramped conditions in which you play. You are on formal, stilted terms even with yourself. If you don't notice you are out there, perhaps no one else will notice either.

All the important players of the early era of the game, dating from 1926 when Dr. Roland Jacobi, a Hungarian attorney, became the first world champion, understood this introspection. For them the game was closer to chess than sport. These players were intellectuals and philosophers. They played cat and mouse with each other, waiting for an opening in the other's argument. Occasionally this mental contest was so evenly matched and exhaustive—in one famous instance it took two hours to decide a single point—that a time limit had to be imposed. But that was rare; mainly such intellectual jousting made for great entertainment, much greater than anything the modern game can offer—where most points are over in three shots—and as a consequence attracted audiences that are not seen today outside the Far East.

One of the darlings of the presponge game was Richard Bergmann, who defended so far back from the table his opponent must have wondered if he'd left the arena; but he wasn't a scrambler; he retrieved balls because he still had something to say. Victor Barna would suddenly unloose an exquisitely lazy backhand, a mere flick of the wrist with which as often as not he would finish the point because he could listen to your nonsense no longer.

That was the shot we all aspired to when I was a boy player in Manchester in the 1950s. It had an argumentative scorn that seemed somehow to belong to literature. Socrates would have enjoyed table tennis, leading your interlocutor on until he comes to see the logical weaknesses in his own game. Marty Reisman's great rival and fellow American champion, Dick Miles, was known to read *Ulysses* between matches and is himself the author of a novel—funny, sad, and sexy—which as far as I know remains shamefully unpublished.

Both Bergmann and Barna, like Jacobi, were from what remained of the Austro-Hungarian Empire. With the exception of the Englishman Fred Perry, every world champion for the first twenty-five years of the game's history came from that crumbling corner of Europe. If table tennis has always been a game that suits people of a quiet, introverted nature—the sad, the melancholic, the disappointed, and the lonely—it is only a short step to understanding why it flowered where it did. Those who played it best in those days were of necessity deracinated solitaries with mournful expressions and quick minds.

Ever since Hiroji Satoh won the World Championship with a sponge bat in 1952, an argument has been quietly advanced for the game he played not being table tennis at all. Once the bat changed from rubber pimples to sponge, some say, the game changed from table tennis to something else. Whatever lawn tennis players think of the technological changes to their equipment over recent years, they go on playing without complaint. Tennis is tennis is tennis. This is an unphilosophical position. Table tennis, true to its dissatisfied, enquiring nature, goes on probing its own status and validity. This is why those of us who play, actually or in our minds, retain such an intense attachment to the game. There is always one more point to replay in our imaginations, always one more question to ask. The game is never over because we cannot decide who really won, and we cannot decide who really won because we are still pondering the nature of victory.

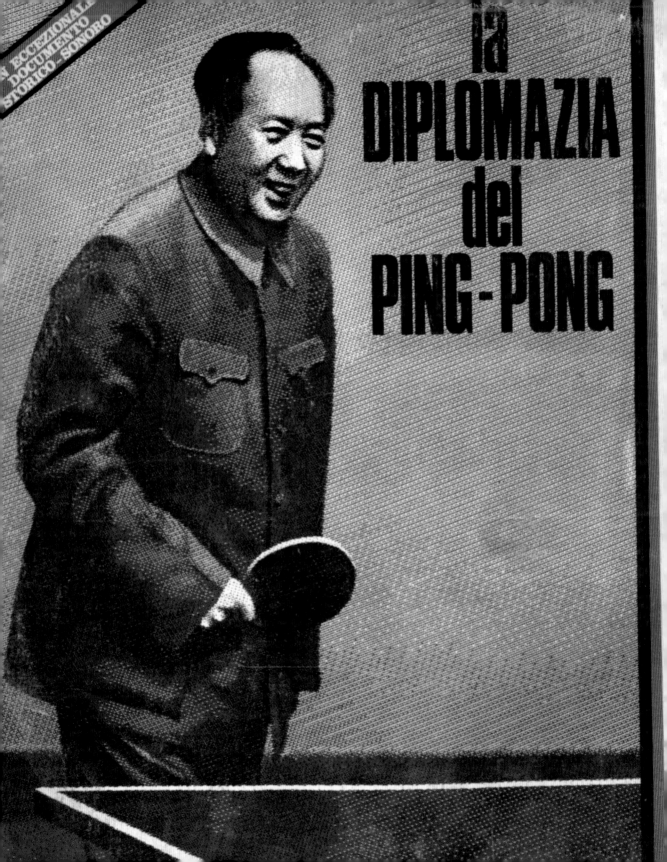

la DIPLOMAZIA del PING-PONG

6

THE GREAT BALL OF CHINA

PING PONG AND
THE CHINESE CENTURY

"Regard a ping pong ball as the head of your capitalist enemy. Hit it with your socialist bat, and you have won the point for the fatherland."

Chairman Mao

China is to ping pong aficionados what the Playboy Mansion is to lifelong onanists: a magical kingdom. The Chinese mainland may be the one place on earth in which ping pong is considered neither a leisure activity nor an ironic distraction for hipsters, but rather the pinnacle of human achievement. Tables litter the cities and countryside. The thwock of rubber on plastic is a familiar and beloved sound, and the nation's history is rich with a tradition of its best and brightest competing to become the stuff of legend.

The relationship between ping pong and China is akin to the love affair

La Cina di Mao (The China of Mao) Long Playing Album, Italy, 1970s.

155

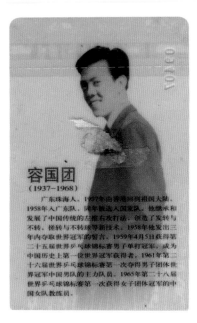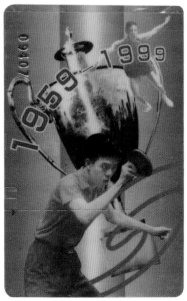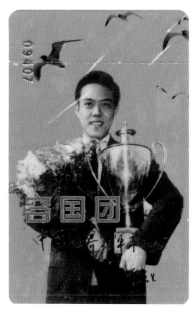

"A spiritual nuclear weapon," says Rong Guotan, China's first world champion. He graces the collectable phone card set celebrating the fortieth anniversary of his 1959 triumph.

between Brad Pitt and Angelina Jolie: two charismatic powers brought together by an unstoppable force, creating something entirely new as they fall fast and hard on the way to greatness. In one case, Brangelina; in the other, sport-transforming world domination. Nine of the world's top ten are Chinese; they have swiped sixteen of the twenty golds ever awarded on an Olympic pedestal. And they don't just dominate under their own flag. Chinese players have spread like chlamydia at a key party, hastily adopting other national identities to fill the ranks of teams the world over. At the last World Championships, a full quarter of the participants representing countries other than China were Chinese-born. Even the mighty USA is not immune: every member of our Olympic team was a naturalized Chinese.

The story of ping pong and China transcends that of a simple tale of a people and their love of a sport. It is a prism through which one can glimpse the nation's extreme makeover from an underperforming centralized state, once known as "the Sick Man of Asia," into a global economic behemoth. The explosive growth of Chinese ping pong has mirrored the country's stop-start

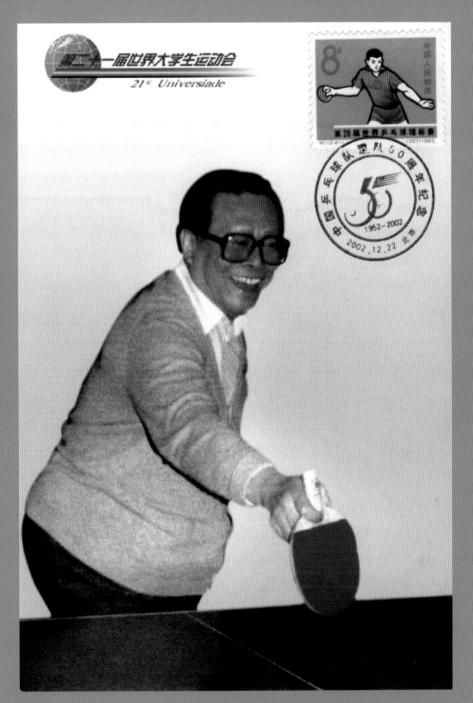

第二十一届世界大学生运动会

21ˢᵗ Universiade

Jiang Zemin, former president of China, on a postcard, circa 2002.

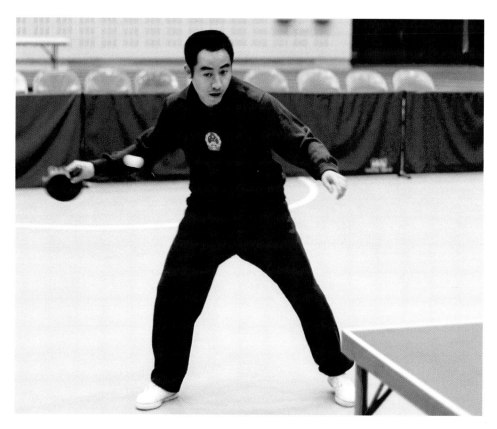

Zhuang Zedong, world champion, politician, and political prisoner.

transformation into a superpower, and its players have been lead actors at every moment of flux—sometimes in the role of inspirational hero, at others, the national punching bag. Ping pong is to China what baseball is to the United States, soccer to Brazil, and *pétanque* is to France: the national sport through which it expresses itself to the world.

Not a bad return for an activity that was originally about as Chinese as General Tso's Chicken, the signature dish of American Chinese cuisine that was actually first cobbled together in a 1970s New York kitchen. Although Sun Tzu's *Art of War* may read in large part like a table tennis manual (Chapter 4: "One defends when his strength is inadequate, he attacks when it is abundant"), ne'er did the sound of a ping or a pong ricochet around the Chinese mainland until the mid-1950s, when the People's Republic of China was

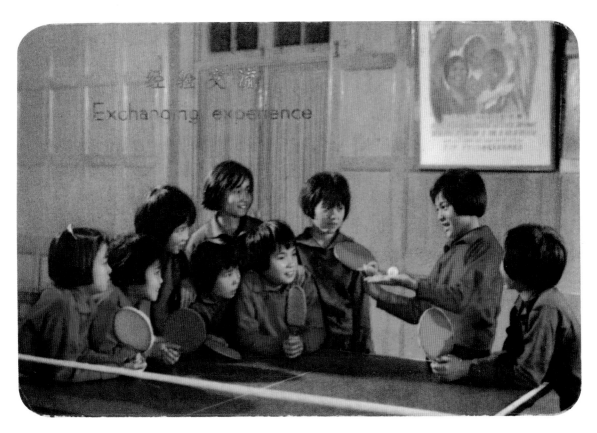

The Exchanging Experience calendar, 1973.

founded, and Mao Zedong adopted his more formidable moniker, Chairman Mao. Mao faced a slew of pressing yet thorny nation-building challenges, agrarian reform and suppressing counterrevolutionaries among them. But near the top of his list was the critical task of defining a national sport. The 1953 decision by the International Table Tennis Federation to become the first sporting body to recognize China made the choice for him. The moment Mao deemed the game to be the nation's priority, the State began to single-mindedly develop a nationwide strategy to ensure the country would soon dominate the world.

Up to this point, the sport was not one that the Chinese had demonstrated any kind of natural proclivity toward. The *New York Times* reported in 1902 that when Foreign Minister Wutingfang was first exposed to the game on

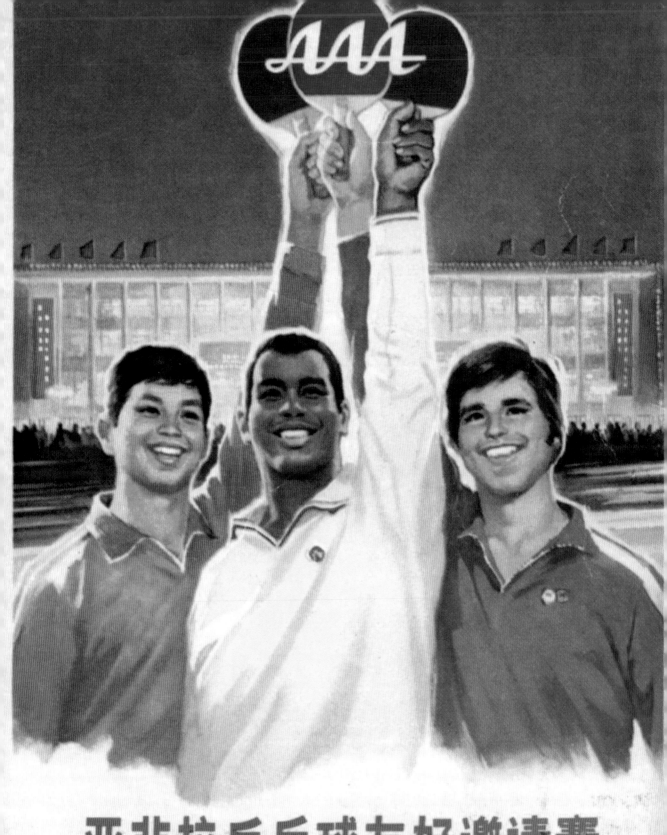

亚非拉乒乓球友好邀请赛

a diplomatic mission to Washington, D.C., he was damning in his critique. "You hit a little ball with a what-do-you-call it. The ball hits the table and the ball says 'ping-pong'; it's a foolish game." But Mao knew better. Ping pong had been predominantly a central European sport, dominated by athletes of the Jewish persuasion; the party leader shrewdly calculated that the Semitic grip would soon be loosened once he let a thousand plastic balls bloom. A legion of bureaucrats was deployed to sweep the nation and test kindergarteners for catlike reflexes and hand-eye coordination. Those demonstrating superior skills were removed from their parents and swiftly dispatched to ping pong academies across the nation where they did little else but train and sleep, tiny cogs in a giant ping pong machine designed to pump out champions.

The sport had another inherent advantage that appealed to Mao: it required little equipment, so it was cheap and easy to spread, in both urban and rural settings. China soon became a magical land in which concrete ping pong tables cropped up everywhere, from public parks and train stations to factory floors. The sport was effortlessly woven into the fabric of Chinese society at both elite and mass levels. Universities began to grant degrees in ping pong, and the game found a natural home at the National Peasant Games, the biggest event on the sporting calendar of the nation's feudal classes, where 3,500 of the most athletic serfs competed in 180 traditional events including the "60 Meter Snatch the Grain and Get It into Storage," "Rice Throwing," and "the Water Carrying Contest to Protect the Seedlings Amidst Drought." Ping pong snuggled comfortably among them, as if its Chinese roots ran deep. It did not take long until every Chinese child could grasp a ping pong bat in a pen hold grip with an air of menace.

Mao was a man obsessed. The multimillion-yuan ping pong machine he created was designed to bring glory to the nation, and he did not have to wait too long for a return on his investment. At the 1959 World Championships in Dortmund, Germany, Rong Guotuan, a former child laborer from the fish market in Nanping Village, Nanping Town, Zhuhai City, used a chop-counter attack to undo his Hungarian opponent, Ferenc Sido, and become China's first world champion in any sport. Rong's victory was spectacular, and not just because the player had to shake a nasty bout of tuberculosis to achieve it. Mao understood that its power surpassed that of a sporting achievement; it was a triumph for the entire nation's self-confidence, and he heralded it as a "spiritual nuclear weapon."

Encouraged, the Great Leader took precious time out from running the country to write a coaching manual that could cement the Chinese stranglehold on the sport. The nation's next champion, Zhuang Zedong, claimed the tome was the inspiration behind the metronomic consistency he used to claim an unprecedented three consecutive world titles between 1961 and 1965. Zhuang developed a unique short-court dual-offensive style, which made him deadly from both the forehand and backhand side of the table, but he was astute enough to underplay his own talent, announcing to the world that the secret to his game was the Great Leader: "I owe my entire table tennis success to the study of Mao's philosophy." This political savvy served Zhuang well; he later was appointed the nation's sports minister.

Ping pong and politics had become so intertwined that when Nixon was searching for an icebreaker to thaw relations with the Chinese Republic, the sport was the obvious medium. After all, what better way could there be for two nations locked in mortal ideological combat to overcome their differences than to play ping pong and kick back like kids in a basement? For the Americans, the diplomatic path was heralded as a stroke of creative genius, but China had used the methodology a number of times before, improving relations with Arab, African, and Latin nations by hosting Friendship Tournaments, with its athletes under strict instructions to throw games at the appropriate times to strengthen political relationships.

What became hailed as a groundbreaking geopolitical achievement began with a missed bus. At the 1971 World Ping Pong Championships, Glenn Cowan, the floppy-haired man-child star of the U.S. team, became separated from the rest of his squad on the trip between hotel and venue and was forced to hitch a ride on the next shuttle. As fate would have it, this bus carried

Glenn Cowan, spreader of good vibes and accidental pioneer of Ping Pong Diplomacy.

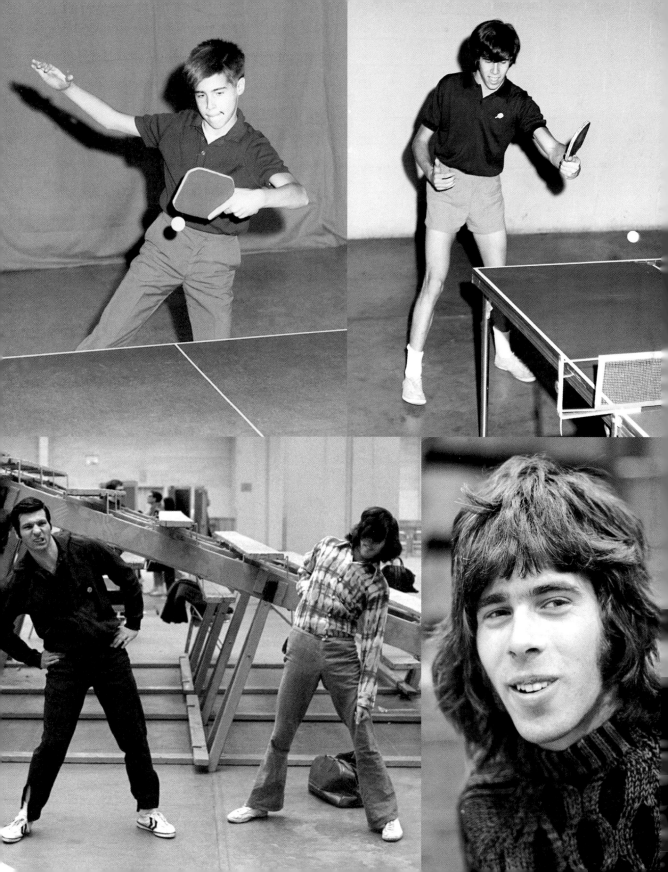

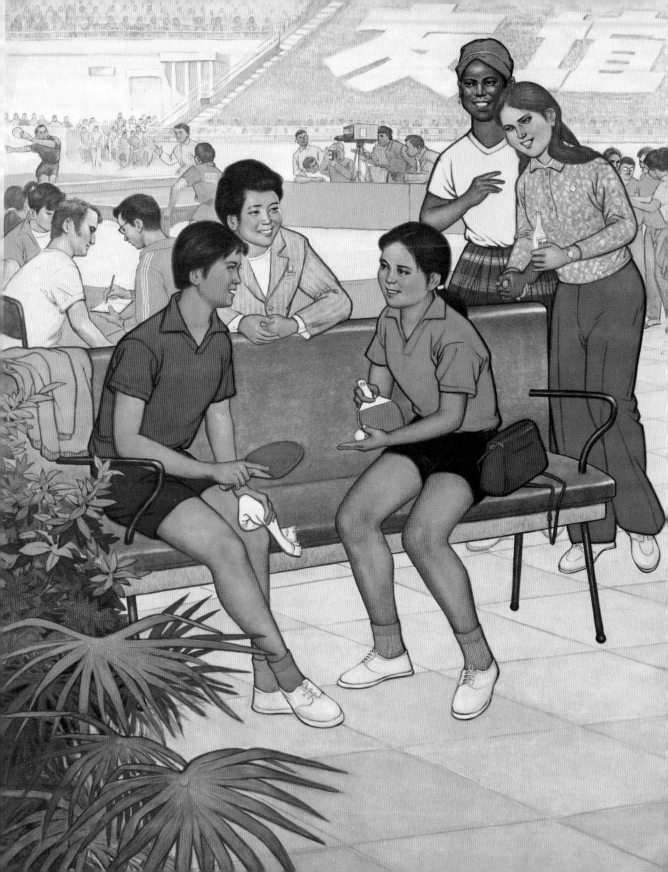

the Chinese team. At first, the Chinese players pretended they could not see the lanky Cowan, terrified they would be punished as spies or traitors once they returned home. But Zhuang was confident enough to break the silence, presenting the American with a brocade silk scarf as a gesture of welcome. The two players alighted to the flashbulbs of paparazzi eager to capture the unprecedented symbol of an American athlete jumping off a Chinese bus. The following day Cowan tracked down Zhuang, eager to return his generosity by presenting him with a gift that summed up the finest America had to offer: a used T-shirt emblazoned with the peace symbol and the phrase LET IT BE. The gift exchange triggered a tumult in the press, which gave Nixon the opening he needed to negotiate with his Chinese counterparts and announce within a week that the United States team would tour China to play in a spirit of "friendship first, competition second."

Cowan proudly led his team on a trip that ultimately laid the groundwork for Kissinger, and then Nixon himself, to follow. The highlight was when the American, ever the free spirit, asked the Chinese prime minister for his thoughts on the hippie movement. The premier did not miss a beat before cryptically replying, "Young people ought to try different things but they should try to find something in common with the great majority." Perhaps the premier's mind was on other matters, such as marketing Double Happiness, the official brand of Chinese ping pong equipment that was launched in the United States in the wake of the trip.

If this was the high point for Chinese ping pong, the nadir was the Cultural Revolution, the national effort to reradicalize a society that was perceived to be slipping into capitalist habits, a task achieved by encouraging students and peasants to wreak revenge on the intellectual classes. Millions were killed, imprisoned, or forced to relocate for reeducation according to the Little Red Book. The national ping pong team was too powerful a national symbol to be left out of the fray, and during the benignly named "Clean up the Class Campaign" they were slandered as a hotbed of anti-Maoist revisionism. Shockingly, Rong Guotuan was among the leading Pongistas who fell victim. In 1968, just nine years after he had triumphed in Dortmund, he committed suicide during Red

Guard torture, leaving behind a suicide note: "I love my honor more than my life." The ping pong diplomat Zhuang survived the bloodshed, only to be discredited a month after Mao died in 1976 for his connections to Mao's widow and her "Gang of Four," as well as for the crime of being rumored to wear a "Swiss-made watch." He was sentenced to four years of solitary confinement in a cramped room, during which his only human interaction was with the guards and interrogators.

A second crisis for Chinese ping pong came from within the game itself: the 1980s rise of Jan-Ove Waldner, a Swede known as the Mozart of Table Tennis. Resplendent with his signature mullet, Waldner was the master of the long rally. Matthew Syed of the *London Times* poetically described his majesty: "His playing narrative is more akin to James Joyce than Jane Austen. Yet like Austen's prose, Waldner's stroke-making is deployed with unrivaled subtlety and grace." His ascension to world champion in 1989 triggered an existential crisis across China, as the entire nation struggled to understand how a tiny country like Sweden, with a mere 10,000 ping pong players, could trump one with over 300 million registered fanatics. Chinese coach Lu Lin was among those mystified, conceding that although Waldner was "born for table tennis, he is an ordinary man off the table tennis court. No girlfriend, unable to drive. Busy with competing and making money, yet leaving his finances to his older brother. Except table tennis he is good at almost nothing."

Waldner's emergence became a watershed for Chinese ping pong and triggered a complete overhaul of the state-run system. Even as the Swede leveraged his superstar status by opening the first meatball/ping-pong-themed restaurant in Beijing, the Chinese ping pong federation adapted to his techniques and began to allow its players to keep a percentage of their prize money, a decision reflecting widespread reforms occurring throughout the country as Deng Xiaoping navigated a path toward a market economy. Unlike older athletes who were forced to claim that their motivation lay in the nation's glory (Zhuang magnanimously claimed his role in ping pong diplomacy was worth the monetary equivalent of "a thousand titles"), the younger athletes remained assets of the state but were now allowed to keep half their winnings.

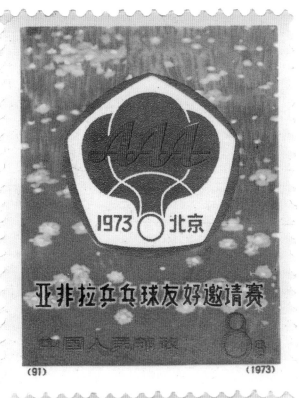

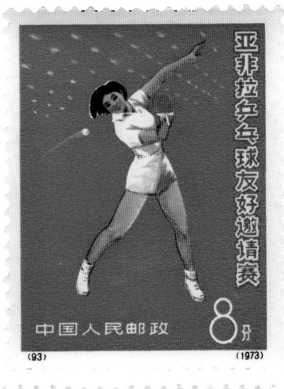

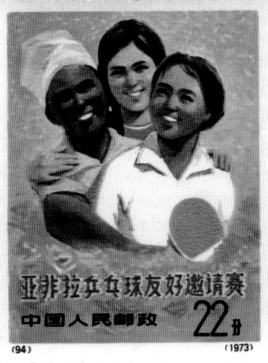

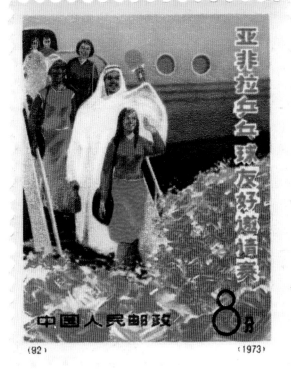

Chinese stamp set celebrating International Friendship tournament, 1973.

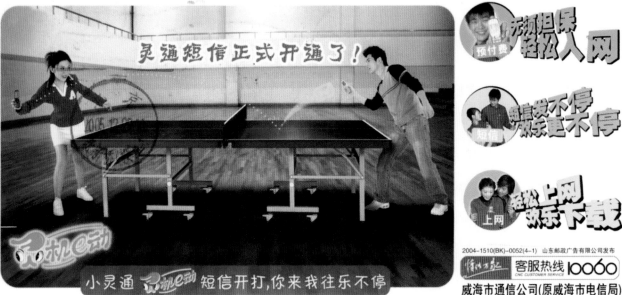

The spoils of this new policy were soon evident. When Wang Nan won the 2000 Olympics women's gold, her traditional old-school reward (in her case, being appointed the delegate from Lianoning Province to the Chinese Party Congress) was augmented by the lucrative contract she received to serve as spokeswoman and poster child for a sanitary towel company. Once the money began to flow, ping pong players became ping pong *playas*. World champion Wang Hao celebrated his 2008 Beijing Olympic gold medal by urinating on the side of a nightclub. After excusing himself in a liquid sense, he excused himself verbally, offering security guards who sought to apprehend him the following explanation: "I am the famous Wang Hao! I am the world champion! Does it matter if I beat you?" (Warning: Don't try that one at home, gentle readers.)

In this brave new world of Chinese ping pong, pissing on the side of buildings was permissible. The only cardinal sin was for team members to woo and court. Four players were dropped from the Athens Olympic team for dating: three women—Li Nan, Bai Yang, and Fan Ying—were sent home to "carry out deep reflection." (For more on this tale of unbridled passion, please see "Forehand Foreplay and the Topspin Seduction," page 72.) Shades of the old regime also reappeared when Chen Qi kicked a chair into the air after losing to fellow countrymen in the China Cup and was promptly sent to the country-side for seven days of reeducation in the northern province of Heibi "to level dirt, weed, and pick cucumbers."

Complacency and loose bladders are not the only threats to ongoing Chinese supremacy. The greatest challenge the players currently face comes from being so damn good that young Chinese are turning away from the sport, their passion dulled by the predictability of the results and the monotonous inevitability of Chinese victory. Television ratings have plummeted and participation rates are on the decline. A young generation who have had their eyes widened by the Internet, video games, and satellite TV have realized that a wide world of sport exists away from the ping pong table. Now that everyone wants to be LeBron (or *Xia-Huang-Di,* the Little Emperor, his Chinese nickname), ping pong has grown stale fast.

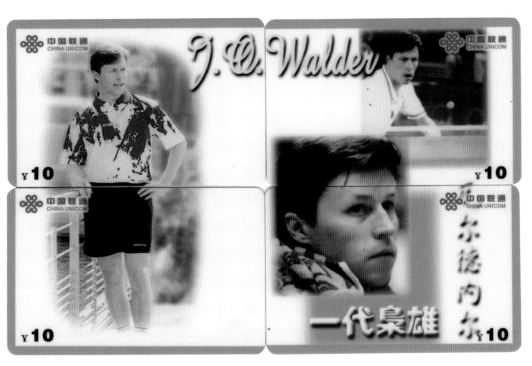

Jan Ove Walder, the Mozart of table tennis, is the face of four China Unicom phone cards.

Change has also occurred at the government level. Repeated glory in the ping pong arena has been tarnished by a growing sense that the rest of the world has given up on the sport. Fueled by the confidence born of economic growth, the Chinese government has expanded its ambition and redirected its resources to defeat the capitalist powers on their own turf. The same methodologies that were once the sole purview of ping pong have been invested in other sports, leading directly to a slew of new role models—Yao Ming on the basketball court, Liu Zige in swimming, and hurdler Liu Xiang.

The hallowed national status of Chinese ping pong is fading fast. If the country's top players want to glimpse their future, they should study the rise and fall of Jacques Secrétin, the greatest *pongiste* the French nation has ever produced. The angular Secrétin became one of the first French champions in any sport when he claimed the World and European titles in the mid-1970s. These achievements were received with rapture by an insecure French nation

A commemorative postcard of the all-conquering Beijing 2008 Olympic team champions.

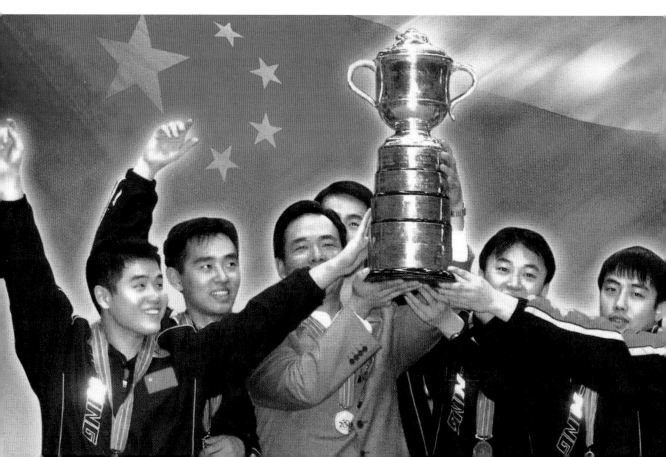

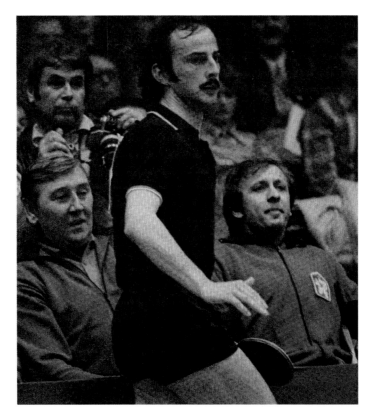

Jacques Secrétin in action.

still deeply traumatized in the wake of World War II. Yet despite the glory of his triumph, Secrétin was unable to shake the embarrassment of his last name, which in French means "like a moron," and the nation replaced him in their affections at the very first opportunity. The moment the French national soccer team reached the semifinals of the 1982 World Cup, Secretin was ejected from the public eye. Today he ekes out a living, augmenting the income he receives from performing in the fringe theater production "The Music Ping Show" by executing ping pong tricks for hire at children's birthday parties. Enjoy urinating against nightclubs while you still can, Wang Hao.

Deutschland, Deutschland über Alles

We have argued that today's Wang Hao may be tomorrow's Jacques Secrétin—lonely, anonymous, condemned to birthday parties and novelty acts. It's a natural progression, certain as the seasons. This cycle raises another question, however—who is tomorrow's Wang Hao? As the Chinese spotlight drifts from ping pong to more superficial pleasures, what nation is prepared to elevate their players to godlike status, free to urinate on any building they please?

The answer may be the birthplace of the übermensch: Germany. The country is currently a second-rate pong power, but their attention to detail and proven commitment to global domination should serve them well. And as the trading cards within attest, a fleet of attractive men and women are already iconic figures among *Tischtennisspielerin*. The propoganda machine is in place, and the players are ready.

The leader of this blitz is the enigmatic Timo Boll. Every German schoolchild fondly remembers those glorious final months of 2002, when Boll defeated Wang Liqin and Kong Linghui and assumed the top spot in the world rankings. After six fragrant months, the Chinese regained their traditional crown, but Boll has continued to nip the heels of greatness, a fixture in the top five.

On the women's side, the brightest stars have just begun to shine, in the persons of the young Solja sisters. Amelie, nineteen, was a runner-up in the World Juniors and is already up to number 9 in the German rankings. Lil' sis Petrissa is close behind, at number 11—and only sixteen years old! Will the Solja name soon ring out alongside Nowitzki, Schrempf, and Blab in the pantheon of Germanic athletic greatness? A nation of Solja soldiers sits poised on the precipice.

JÖRG ROSSKOPF

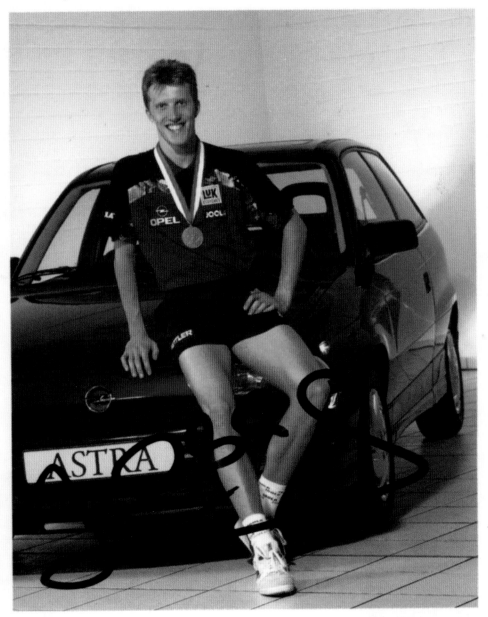

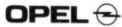

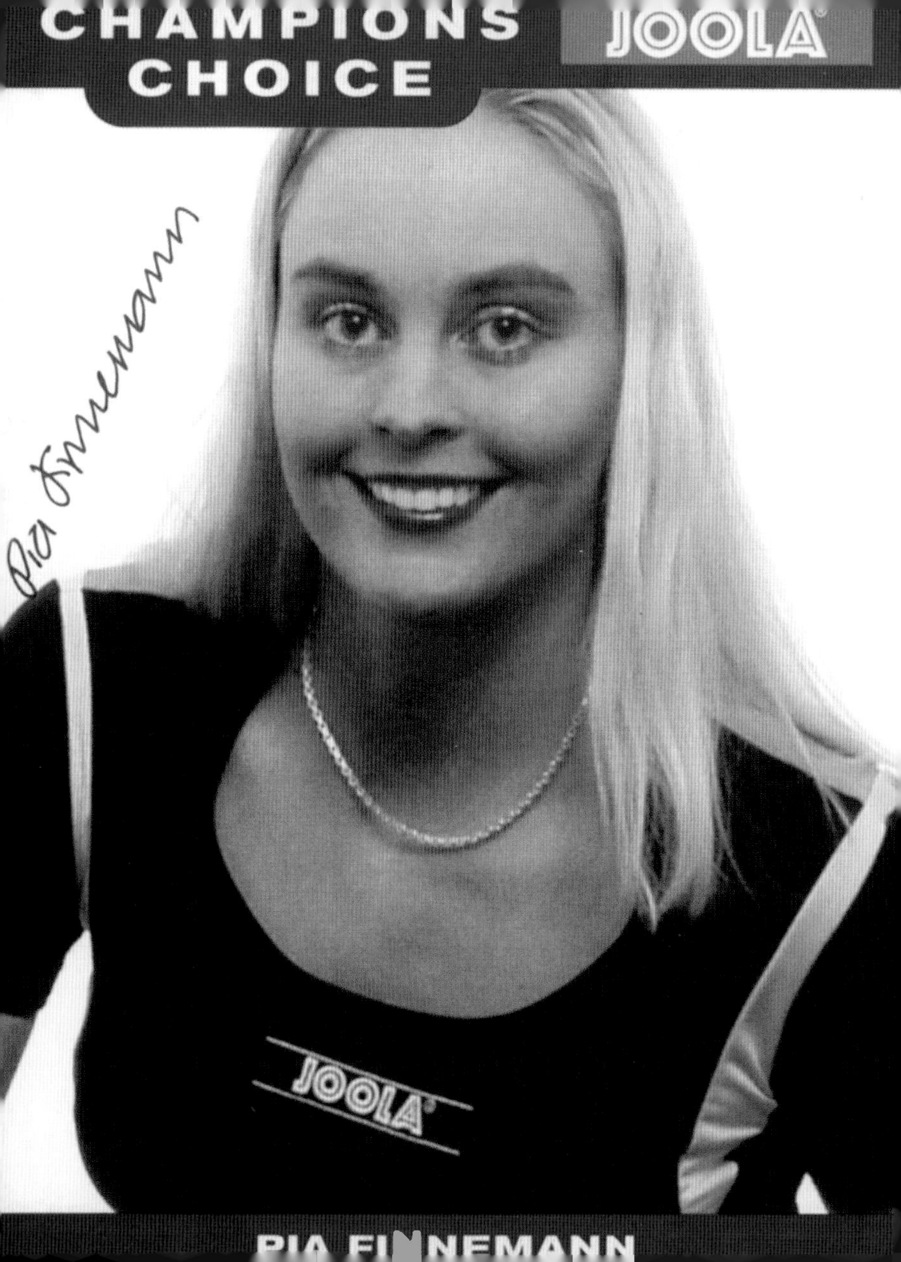

CHAMPIONS CHOICE JOOLA

JOOLA

PIA FINNEMANN

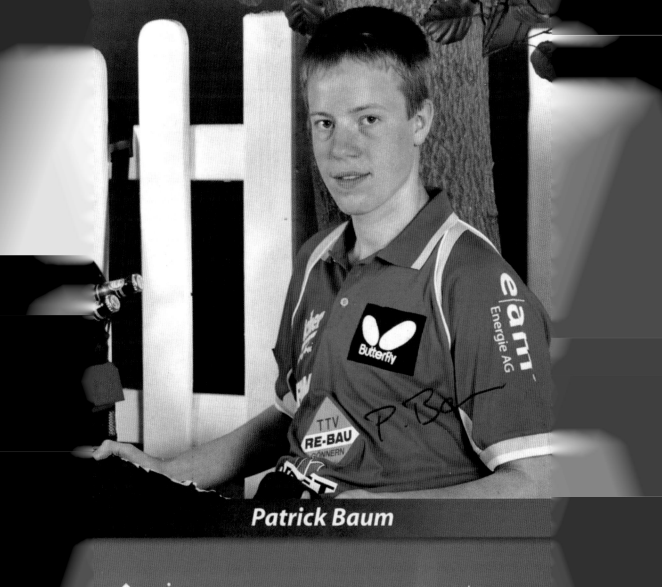

Patrick Baum

        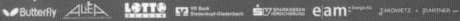   

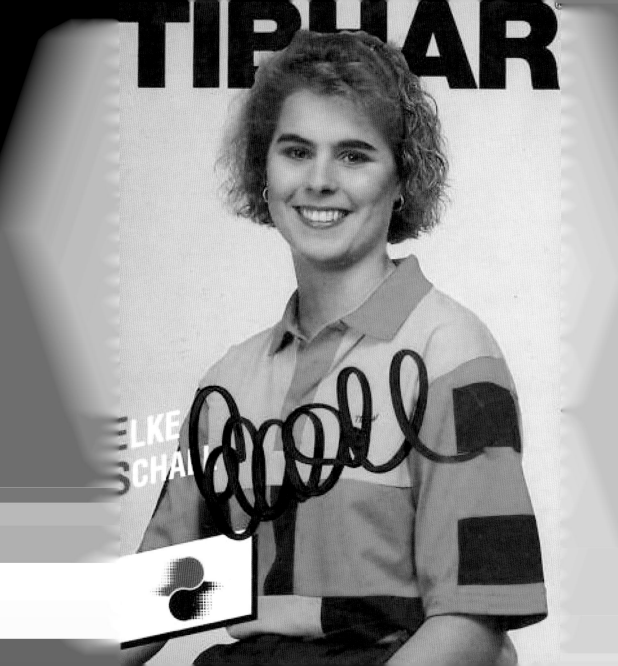

TIBHAR

ELKE
SCHA

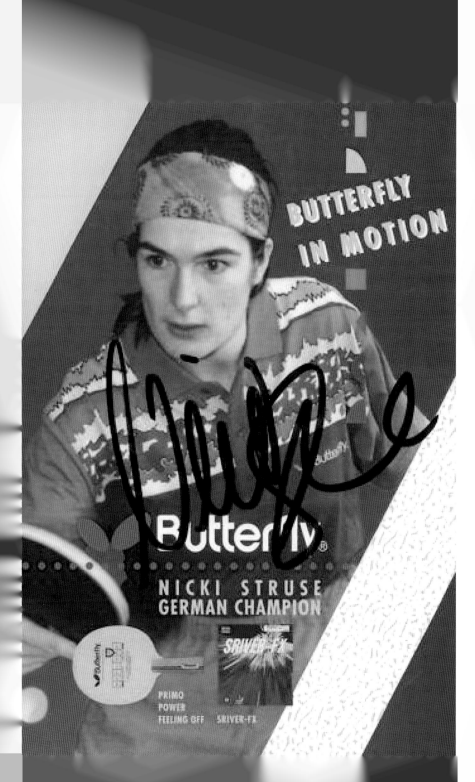

BUTTERFLY
IN MOTION

Butterfly®

NICKI STRUSE
GERMAN CHAMPION

SRIVER-FX

PRIMO
POWER
FEELING OFF   SRIVER-FX

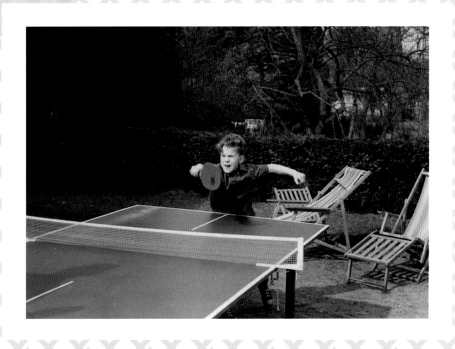

ZEN AND THE ART OF FORGETTING

BY STARLEE KINE

Somewhere tangled up in the horrible jumble that was my fourteenth year lives a hazy, lazy memory of a class trip to the Richard Nixon Library in Yorba Linda, California. Richard Nixon and I spent our childhoods in nearby Whittier, although not at the same time. Forty years before I was born, he was being booed off the stage of his high school's production of *The Aeneid* alongside his first real love. (It didn't last—she hated his mood swings.)

I remember the weight of large, foamy headphones over my ears, whispering censored snippets of the Watergate recordings to me like a busybody up to no good. I remember I was spending a lot of time with a boy named Trevor, my fifth true love, stepping on the backs of his shoes every chance I got. I remember being corralled into a little carpeted room, twenty or so classmates on the floor, forty or so crossed legs. Our teacher tells us we are lucky, there's a very special guest there that day. Fifteen or so necks craning to see. Five or so pens doodling on the soles of ten or so sneakers. We hope for someone famous. We hope for someone good. We hope for Alan Thicke or Michael

Jackson or Ricky Schroder. A man enters, wearing a suit. He has a flattop haircut, similar to Trevor's. His name is H. R. Haldeman. He has something important to tell us. We hope he wants to tell us about how he is not the real special guest. We hope he wants to talk about his best friend, whom he brought with him, Belinda Carlisle or Alex Trebek or Alf.

Our smiling teacher says, "Mr. Haldeman used to work for President Nixon. You know how you feel when you do something bad like hit your little sister on the arm? You know how you feel sort of okay about it unless your little sister runs and tells your mom and then you get in trouble and then you feel worse? That's what happened with Mr. Haldeman and President Nixon. They did something bad and got in trouble for it and that made them feel bad."

H. R. Haldeman, tall, suited, trying to figure out how to start. He wants us to know that President Nixon did a lot of good, too. "Raise your hand if you've ever been to China." Forty or so hands attached to forty or so arms continue to dangle awkwardly from adolescent bodies that are shooting up in crazy ways. Not one of these hands is raised. In fifth grade I chose the purple crayon to color China in on the world map I was given in class. That feels like it should count for something. I raise just my index finger, so that only I can see. H. R. Haldeman pauses, chews his lip, thinks about his next segue. He looks up, inspired. "Raise your hand if you've ever played ping pong." Thirteen or so hands shoot up. One hand, mine, shoots up, shoots down, shoots back halfway up.

We didn't have a ping pong table in our house. My family didn't have a basement, which I've been told is where they are usually kept. They are also sometimes kept in garages, but we didn't have one in there either. That's where we kept moving boxes full of belongings that we never unpacked. It's possible that a ping pong table was in one of those boxes, in pieces, a prefab home to spiders who would've preferred the cool pockets of a pool table but still were grateful for what they had. I have often wondered how different my life would've turned out had I grown up in a ping-pong-playing family. I imagine these families having fights and then heading to the ping pong table to cool off.

I know these houses when I see them. I was at one the other day. A mom and a dad and their three little kids. The daughter took me out to the garage by the hand. She wanted me to teach her how to play. We failed to get a rally going, and she quickly grew bored. "How about if we play with this bottle cap, instead?" she said, scouring the ground for trash. "Or this bubble blower. Or this piece of fluff. How about this bit of rotten plum?" Almost all of them, whether limping or soaring, managed to make their way over the net. The piece of fluff, friendless and alone, was the only holdout.

"Did you know," H. R. Haldeman continues, "that President Nixon was the only lifetime honorary member of the United States Table Tennis Association?" We sense we are being fed information, data. We fear we will be tested on this later. Forty or so eyes, plus two from our teacher, begin to glaze over. H. R. Haldeman switches into storytelling mode. He says, "There once was a ping pong player, named Glenn Cowan, who missed his bus. This was in Japan, quite far from his house. There was no way he could have just walked home. He got on another bus, one full of Chinese ping pong players. The most popular one, named Zhuang Zedong, came and sat next to him. The whole bus gasped, the same way you would gasp if the most popular kid in your class suddenly sat down next to the least popular kid." At this, the most popular kid in our class punched the least popular kid on the arm, hard. "Zhuang Zedong reached in his bag and pulled out a lovely silkscreen of a mountain. Glenn Cowan reached in his bag and turned up only a comb. 'I can't give you a comb' he said, 'I wish I could give you something. But I can't.' At the bus stop, the press was waiting. They snapped picture after picture of the two players together, Zhuang probably secretly wishing the whole time he had that comb in order to fix up his hair. In any case, though, that's how Ping Pong Diplomacy was born."

For the first and only birthday of mine that Trevor was around to celebrate, he reached into his backpack and pulled out a bottle of perfume, a quarter full. He had found it under the sink in his parents' bathroom. It made me seem both older and younger when I wore it. It smelled the way little kids who wore glasses looked.

My grandmother still has a Polaroid of Trevor and me at a school dance, framed up nice, prominently displayed. Besides my grandfather, Trevor's photo is the only picture of a male in the whole house. Even at ninety-five, my grandmother is swift with her scissors, cutting out of the shot anyone she perceives to have broken our hearts. (My sister's wedding album is a mess of jagged-edged pictures of her standing all alone in her lovely gown.) Trevor was also the only boyfriend of mine who I wasn't completely crazy about—in the photo I am standing on tiptoes in order to fake-throttle him, Homer Simpson–style—and there have been nights when I've slept with his photo under my pillow, hoping to understand what my grandmother saw in him that I never did.

In college my little sister went off to Madrid to pretend to study. She ran through the streets eyes shut, hair streamed, youth flaunted. One day she came up against a wall that was actually the chest of a man named Franzi. He was the fifth-best ping pong player in all of Spain. I remember a breathless conversation with my sister over the phone, each word like a coin out of our pockets and thus having to be worthy and right. She chose to spend her money on a description of the way Franzi brushes his teeth. His hand held the toothbrush as though it were a paddle, she told me, with the fifth-greatest of finesse. It came as no surprise that this was what my sister chose to focus on. The youngest of the cousins, we'd grown up studying the mangled photos at our grandmother's house long before we were featured in them. Our first crushes were on disembodied hands. So naturally it was a hand that my sister started with now, slowly working outward from there.

H. R. Haldeman reaches into his inside coat pocket and pulls out an index card. Written on it are words from a speech Richard Nixon gave. When he begins to speak, he doesn't look down at the card once. He already knows the words. "We know, too, that in the course of your contest there will be winners and losers. But there is one big winner, and that is more important than who wins a match in table tennis. The big winner, because of this people-to-people contact that you are initiating between our two peoples, will be friendship between the people of the United States and the people of the People's Republic of China."

Ten years or so passed. I moved into and out of a half-dozen or so apartments. I became a writer. I did many or so dishes. I was accepted into the kind of artist residency that had cabins and fireplaces and murmurings of affairs. Just before it began, my heart was broken so thoroughly that my grandmother's scissors moved of their own accord in the drawer where they were kept. They swished back and forth like a napping toddler kicking off his covers.

Once I got to the residency, pretty much all I did was play ping pong. At first I barely had enough strength to hold the paddle. I'd have to rest between swings. I'd faint after a particularly strenuous rally. Sometimes the ping pong ball would ping pong on the table in front of me and I'd fall into a trance and just let it do its thing.

For the first month, I couldn't sleep without dreaming about things that weren't true anymore. I'd wake up traumatized and stumble into the common area. There I would perform my daily ritual: pressing my cheek against the ping pong table for as long as it took to calm down. Lots of people had daily rituals there. It was that kind of place. A Buddhist composer named Koji would meditate every morning and play ping pong every afternoon. My daily ritual kept getting in the way of his daily ritual, and so he suggested we combine. He began to teach me lessons of the Buddha as the game nursed me back to health. He told me not to worry about my backhand, that what I needed was to be more straightforward. He told me I didn't have to keep bouncing around so much, that sometimes staying still was more active than movement. He told me the point wasn't to win, and I wanted to whisper back, I know, Koji, I know, the point is that China loves me even if my true love does not. One million or so games later, I finally went to sleep and dreamt I was floating through space.

"I want to talk about heartbreak," H. R. Haldeman says. "I loved him like a brother." He feels more like one of us now, closer to our size. From the back, because of his hair, we can pretend he is one of the boys. We can pretend we have stared at that back of a head our whole lives. The least popular kid is curled in a ball, asleep, drooling on the carpet. One by one, the rest of us take turns drawing on his face with a marker, obscuring his tear-stained cheeks with mustaches and stars and lines from our favorite songs.

Boy's Own
PAPER

JOHNNY LEACH
– WORLD CHAMPION

SEE PAGE 24

BRITAIN'S GREAT CYCLE SHOW
– in this issue

7

VELOUR COUTURE

THE WANING AND WAXING OF PING PONG STYLE

The novelties of one generation are only the resuscitated fashions of the generation before last.

George Bernard Shaw

The 1990s were treacherous years for lovers of ping pong couture. Along with acid-washed jeans, harem pants, and mustaches, the sport's tight shorts and polo chic were left to languish, exposed to the ridicule of empty-headed fickle followers of fashion. But the truly stylish knew they were a sleeping giant of panache, albeit one made of 100 percent polyester. As couture visionary Bruce Oldfield observed, "Fashion is more usually a gentle progression of revisited ideas," and this was never truer than with ping pong. After years of ostracism, the sport's style has recently been rediscovered, and the shorts/long socks/tight shirt combinations it inspired have returned to their rightful status as iconic staples of American fashion.

This sartorial journey from ugly duckling to swan has not always been easy. Ping pong's Paleolithic ages were the early years of the twentieth century, when the sport's look was constricted by the formal dictates of the era.

"Johnny Leach, world champion, man of style, in *Boy's Own Paper*, 1949."

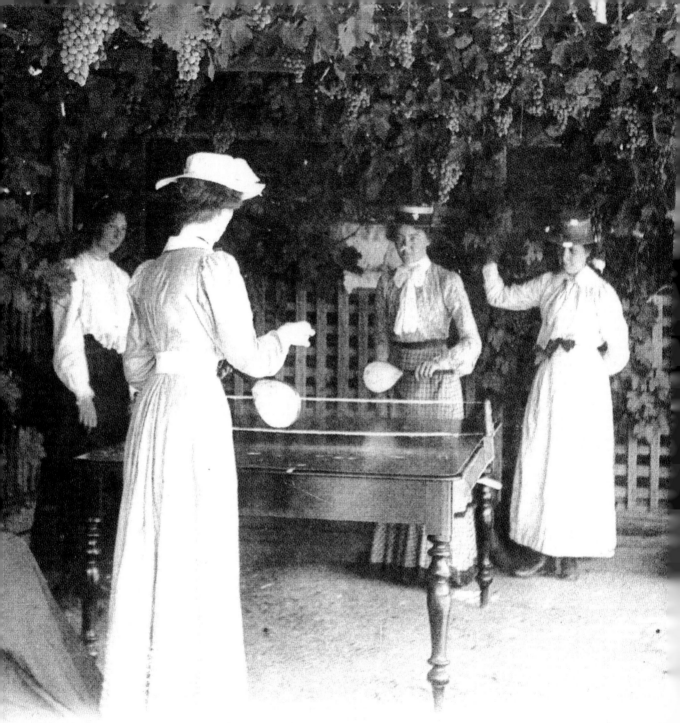

PING PONG UNDER THE VINES. S. A.

Full-length flannels on display in this 1902 postcard.

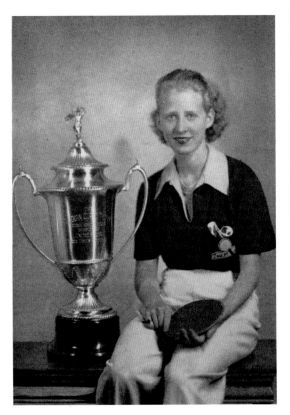 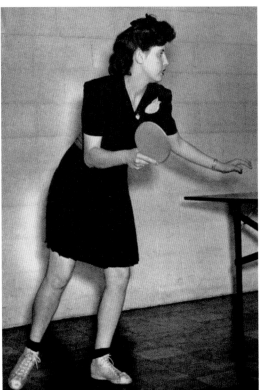

Women go sports-casual, 1950s.

Clothes and performance were yet to be interlinked, and female competitors were especially handicapped. Indeed, players often found their attire more of a challenge than their opponents, as they were expected to take to the table trussed up in heavy full-length flannel dresses, occasionally set off by fur and bustle, with corsets required. The 1902 British champion, a Mrs. Holbrook, dispensed practical fashion pointers as she urged the fairer sex to avoid wearing trains "as in the course of a keen game that form of skirt will surely be stepped on which cannot fail to unsteady the balance somewhat. Moreover it will in all probability injure the skirt, the knowledge of which injury will not tend to help the player to maintain the equilibrium of her temper which has already been sorely tried by the loss of an important stroke."

The prevailing style for gentlemen was long, pleated pants accompanied by a formal shirt or blazer; their minds may have been on ping pong, but

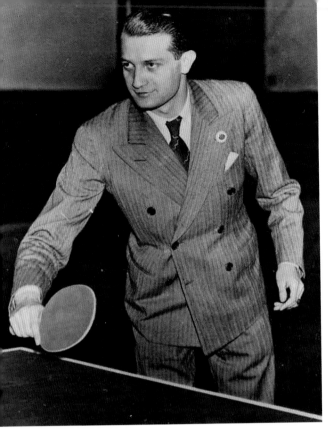
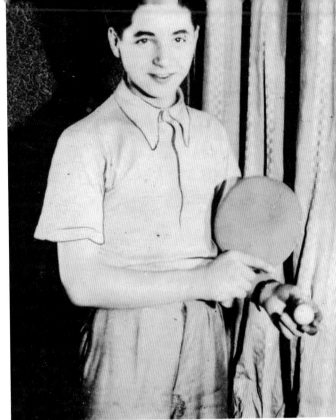
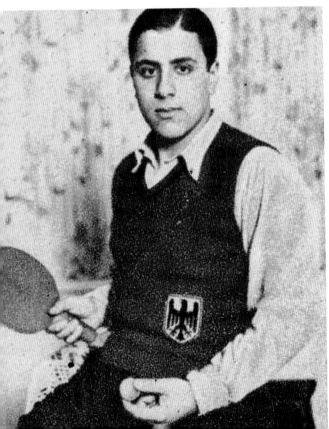
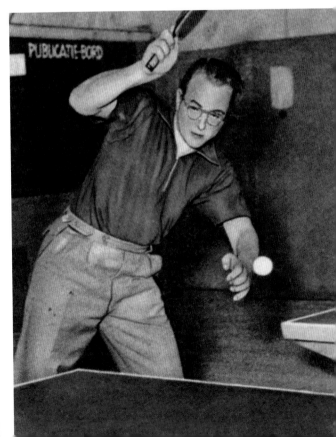

their look said Sunday best. The legendary Victor Barna, who won a record twenty-two world championships titles in the 1930s courtesy of his signature backhand flick, was photographed spraying shots around the table in a dapper double-breasted suit. Barna set the bar high; few were blessed with his innate sense of style. One female player was sufficiently perturbed by what she considered to be slipping sartorial standards to dispatch an anonymous letter to the editor of an English table tennis journal, under the nom de plume "Sartorial": "The menfolk—oh dear—dirty shoes, dirty creased flannels and worst of all, multi-colored braces. It is surely within their means to keep shoes white and trousers creased . . . to emulate Barna . . . in this manner as well as in actual play."

Change was blowing in the wind, though, and it came from the sport's lesser sister, tennis. In the wake of the World War I, feisty Frenchwoman Suzanne Lenglen scandalized Wimbledon by taking the court clad in only a "flimsy and revealing calf-length cotton frock." More shocking: she was hatless, having had the temerity to wear her hair in a band so she could actually see what was going on. It took eight more years before her bare-head antics caught on and ten before the American Alice Marble (who went on to become an associate editor of *Wonder Woman*) was plucky enough to don shorts.

World War II changed everything. Aside from crushing the fascist threat, one of the most significant outcomes of the hostilities was emancipating women from the shackles of sporting formality. Californian tennis star Gussie Moran led the way, donning a Teddy Tinling-designed dress for Wimbledon, which was so short that her ruffled, lace-trim knickers were intentionally and permanently on display. When she served, photographers would battle for position, lying belly-down on the court to sneak upskirt shots that sent shock waves around the globe. Society was forced to adapt to the radical notion that the primary purpose of sporting garb was to enhance athleticism as opposed to maintain modesty. But for some this remained a heretical notion, a hard habit to shake. "Letters to the Editor" pages persisted as the ping-pong-style battleground between the sexes, as one man expressed his distaste after attending a recent tournament at which "a large minority of the women entrants

Top left and right: Formal stylings: Victor Barna, world champion, 1933; H. Lurie, English junior champion and hairdresser, 1935. *Bottom left and right:* Madjargoglou, German champion; Cor Du Buy, Dutch champion, 1937.

were prepared at a moment's notice to transfer themselves to the beach."

But the genie was out of the bottle. Textile technology and mass production were evolving rapidly, America was entering the synthetic age, and a blizzard of inventions indelibly changed ping pong fashion forever, cementing its classic style as a combination of nylon, elastic, comfort, and panache. The addition of color was the first revolution. Ping pong gear had hitherto been almost entirely white to maintain the fiction that humans in general, and women in particular, did not sweat when engaged in athletic pursuit. A London-based sports store, Alec Brook, Ltd., set itself up as a table tennis emporium offering rayon shorts in every shade, including "Sky, Brick, Grey, and Nigger."

The development of new materials encouraged the design of bold new designs. For instance, consider sweatbands. Greek Olympians may have been the first to wrap their hair in wreaths, but the look was not popularized until 1921, when Carl. M. Tipograph utilized terry cloth to soak up the sweat produced by arduous activity. The look was popularized on the heads and wrists of ping pong players, early pioneers some forty years before Bruce Springsteen made the look street-legal.

Another fashion revolution in which pongeurs were early adopters was the advent of sweat suits. In the 1920s, Dr. Oliver Schofield, a British sprinter who went on to invent the electric blender, had the idea of donning a loose-fitting tailored outfit over his shorts to stay warm before a race. The use of velour allowed the suit to combine a luxurious texture with the stretch critical to any athlete. Ping pong teams soon made them standard issue, although some stars found them garish. Frank Gee, a top player of the 1950s and a style traditionalist, was not pleased by the English team's sweat suit he was forced to don when representing the nation. "I consider the word *England* across the back to be unnecessary and beggaring."

As the century progressed, ping pong and style became as one, a vision of synthetic beauty that resonated far beyond the table. First the polo, shorts, and long socks that cloaked the bodies of high-performance masters were adopted as a virtual uniform by middle-aged American tourists on cruises around the world. Next, Olivia Newton John appropriated the look and brought it to millions of followers during the gym boom of the mid-1970s. Then the break dancing explosion of the early 1980s spread sweat suits to both African Americans and suburban teens. The style's appeal began to become overexposed. The zippered nylon sweat suit—a sea foam, mauve, or peach top matched with loose-fitting pants tailored at the waist—became ever present in suburbs and at airport departure gates across the country; wobblebottoms packed our public spaces clad in velour from head to foot. By the 1990s, the look had been written off as the "number one fashion disaster" by a United Kingdom pollster.

Ladies — look your loveliest to Win

★

by

Pinkie Barnes

(popular England & Surrey Star)

★

with a P.S. for men

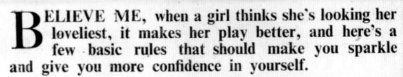

BELIEVE ME, when a girl thinks she's looking her loveliest, it makes her play better, and here's a few basic rules that should make you sparkle and give you more confidence in yourself.

An actress would never dream of appearing on a strongly lit stage without sufficient make-up, but I have often seen quite attractive faces look pale and drawn under the strong, white T.T. lights, when just a few deft touches would have made all the difference.

Yes, quite unashamedly, this is an article about the Art of Looking Your Best, with a few words at the end for critical males.

Don't imagine that the hints I'm going to give you will make you look like a West End mannequin. All you need to know is something about preparations to use, how to apply them, and how to choose colours to tone with your clothes.

The basis of all good looks is a clear, spotless skin, and there's nothing like the vigorous exercise of T.T. to help remove impurities from the skin. Every time you perspire you're doing that very thing. The dust raised while you're playing, however, mixes with perspiration, so you want to make sure to cleanse the skin carefully after an evening's T.T. and ensure that the opened pores do not get clogged.

The golden rule for all skin care is three simple steps :

CLEANSING : STIMULATING : NOURISHING.

Beauty preparations are specially made for different types of skin. I've found that most T.T. players have either dry or normal skins. In my own case (normal) I find a good emollient cleansing cream (first step) followed by a mild skin lotion (second step) and then a rich skin food suit me admirably. I have, of course, my own favourites. There is also one called Milky Cleanser which is perfect for a quick clean-up.

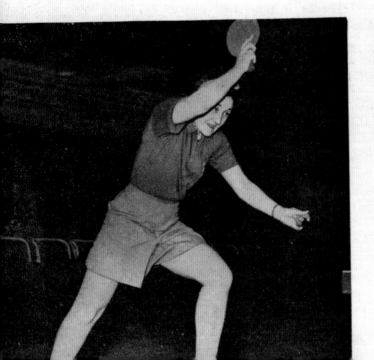

No sports woman in her senses would use a heavy make-up. Use a light powder foundation, preferably a lotion. I particularly recommend Blustery Weather Lotion, which can be used as a powder foundation, hand lotion or a defence against chaps. (Don't get me wrong ; I mean the bad weather variety). It's made by a famous house, is reasonably priced, and you'll like it immediately you see it.

Always choose a face powder that tones with your complexion. Get a light-weight powder because a heavy one goes streaky if you get hot.

Incidentally, I'm all for using a little rouge. You don't often start to colour up until the end of the first set and it's first impressions that count. Without going into the technical details for the various face shapes, I can tell you to bring the rouge up near your eyes, towards the temples. This lessens the sunken look caused by strong lights. Cream rouge will stay on better

(Concluded on opposite page)

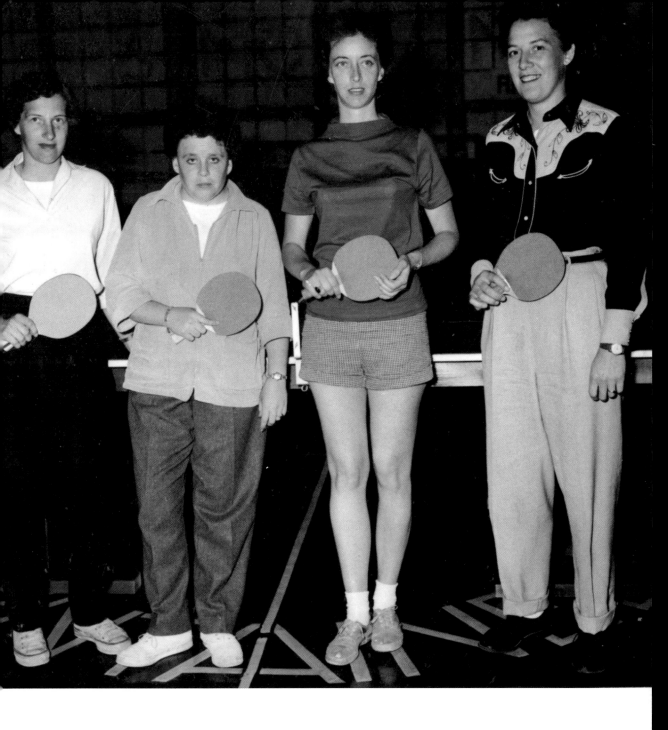

Left: Pinkie Barnes articulates a basic set of rules for ladies style in *Table Tennis* magazine, 1947.

Above: Four anonymous ladies roundly ignore it, circa 1967.

Table Tennis Review

Vol. 7   No. 2

WINTER ISSUE 1952   1/-

Founded by
ARTHUR WAITE
Ex-International

★

ENGLAND

versus

FRANCE

**REPORT
AND RESULTS**

★

TOURNAMENTS
Reports and Results

★

RANKING LISTS

★

Contributors include
**ALEC BROOK
SAM KIRKWOOD**
plus our regular
Correspondents

★

Cover Portrait :
JACKIE KOEHNKE
All-American
1952 Midget Girl Champion

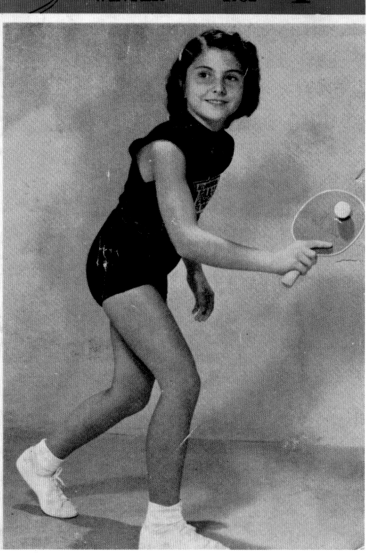

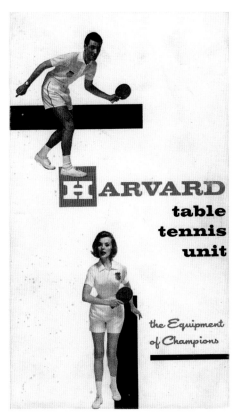

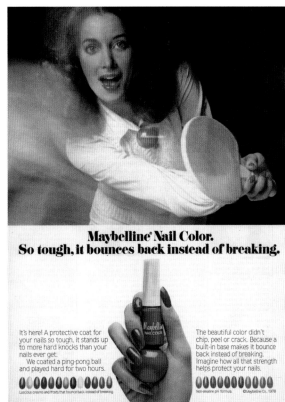

Left: Harvard table tennis unit, 1950s. *Right:* Maybelline nail color advertisement in *Teen* magazine, July 1979.

And so began the lean years. The 1990s were a time of shame, ridicule, and derision, and the elements of ping pong style were cast into the shadows. The *New York Times* described the sport's look as if it was stuck inside the fashion equivalent of a 1970s rec room: "Table-tennis champions compete in baggy shirts tucked into elastic waistbands. The shorts are so loose that players sometimes hike them up during matches, creating the effect of a saggy diaper." This was a period of introspection for the renowned ping pong manufacturers such as Joola and Butterfly, who began to experiment with new microfibers, believing salvation lay in the next great synthetic material. But they need not have worried: ping pong style was soon to be rediscovered. Like an ugly-duckling star at the end of a teen movie who only has to remove her spectacles and shake out her hair to transform herself from bookish nerd

At the ready: Jackie Koehnke, All-American Midget Girl Champion, 1952.

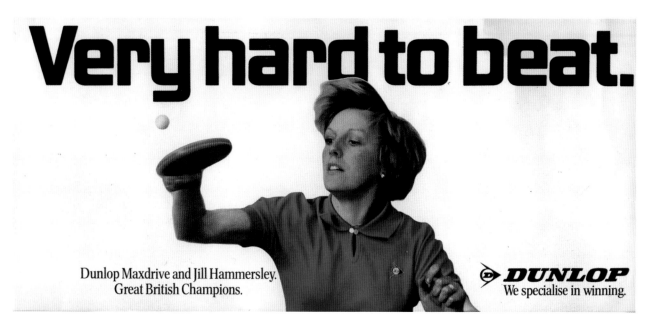

Very hard to beat.

Dunlop Maxdrive and Jill Hammersley.
Great British Champions.

◈ **_DUNLOP_**
We specialise in winning.

Jill Hammersley, British champion and fantasy figure in the minds of a generation of English public school boys in the 1970s.

to object of desire, ping pong would once again become a thing of beauty.

The man who began this revolution was Dov Charney, the self-styled hustler garmento who built the American Apparel brand by blatantly raiding the 1970s and 1980s. Charney understood that the elements of ping pong style—velour, terry cloth, and polyester—were akin to carbon buried deep below the seabed, out of sight perhaps, but far from idle. In his hands, they metamorphosed into beautiful diamonds, finding their way onto the bodies of teen girls on college campuses nationwide, mixing ping pong magic with a pair of Chuck Taylors and some selvage skinny jeans. Yet the powers that be in the ping pong world still did not believe. In 2009, having failed to attract more fans to the sport by experimenting with both the scoring system and the size of tournament balls, the International Table Tennis Federation threw the ping pong equivalent of a Hail Mary pass. Vice president Claude Bergeret, a Frenchwoman, urged players on the ladies tour to ditch the traditional ping pong look and sexy up their style because "*ne pas être habillée comme un sac à patates.*" (You do not want to be dressed like a sack of potatoes.) The French

Kjell Johansson, Lagos Open champion, 1978. Unknown polo pioneer. A gallery of male function over fashion. Daniel Seemiller, 1992. Carl Prean, English champion, 1980s.

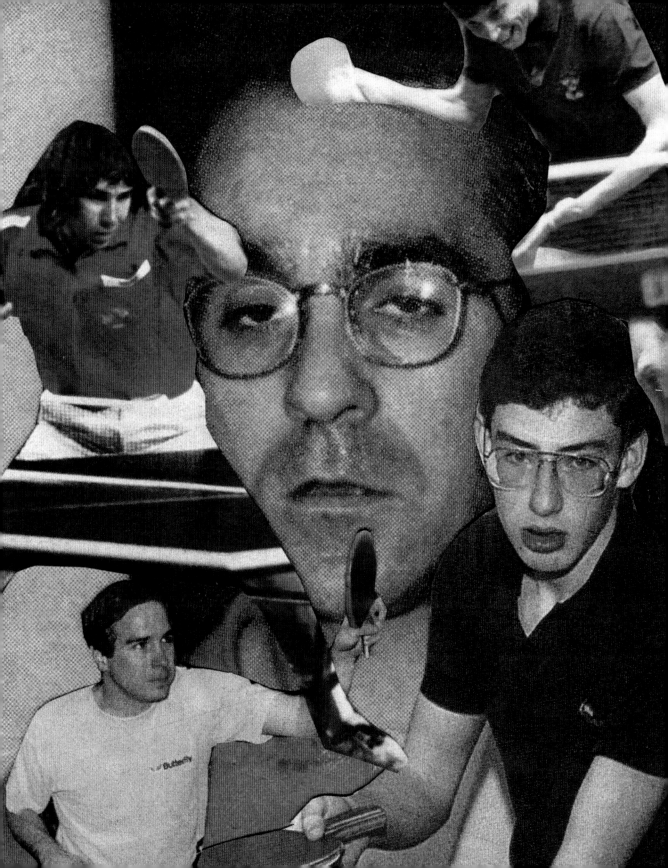

have been responsible for so many misguided opinions in their time that they gave the world the word *faux pas*, but Bergeret's quote must be up there with Marie Antoinette's "Let them eat cake!" As Charney understood so lucratively, ping pong's greatest stylistic strength is its innate authenticity.

Ping pong is not cool, because all cool is temporary—a fleeting fad. Ping pong style is timeless, the sporting equivalent of the little black dress. The designer who appreciates this above all others is Andy Spade, who grew up playing the sport from fifth grade on in the rec rooms of Scottsdale, Arizona. His tastemaking ethos is based in appreciating the unappreciated. In his words, "I originally imagined Jack Spade as a club anyone could get into," and so

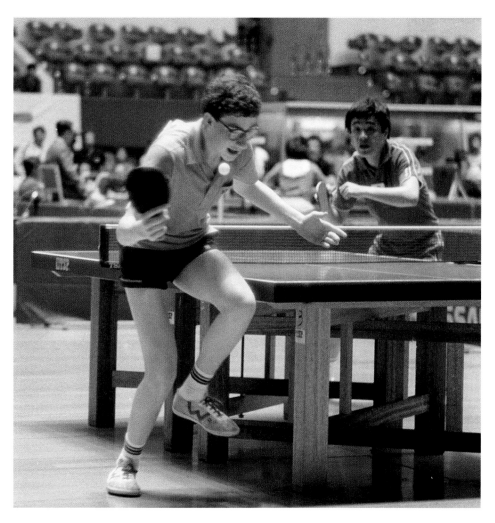

Carl Prean displaying a service technique so deadly the ITTF had to change their rules . . . twice.

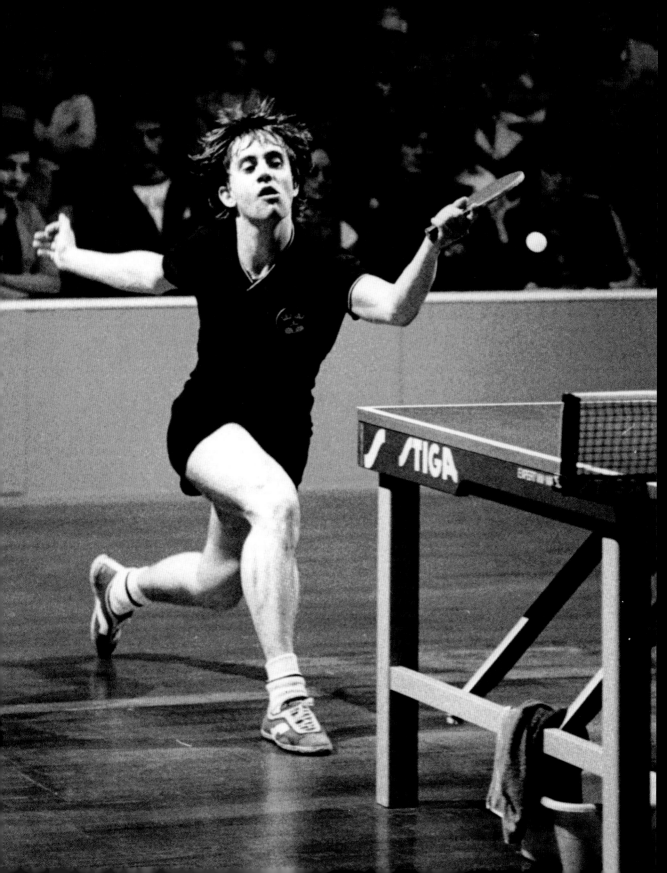

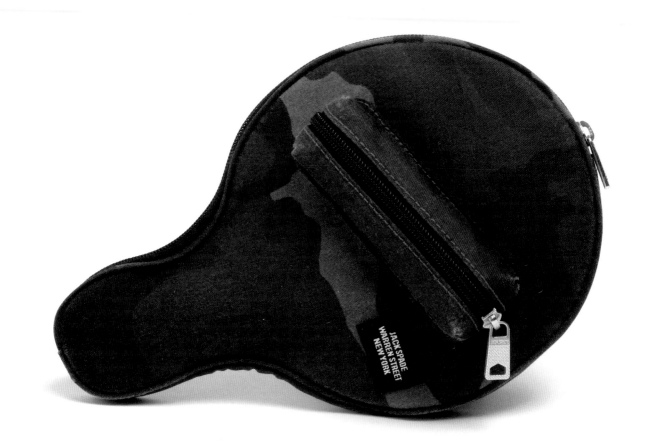

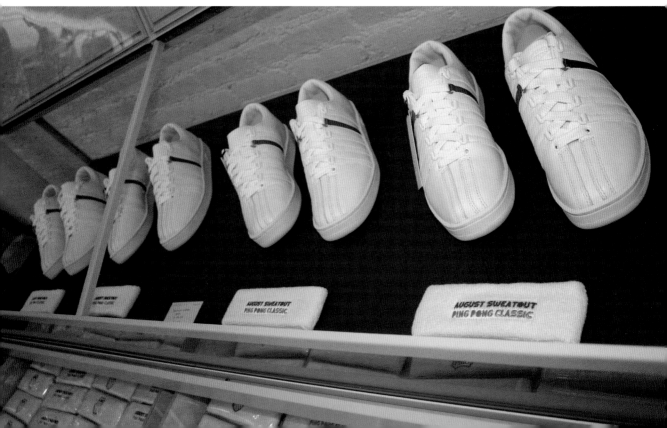

ping pong was a comfortable fit, alongside frog dissection kits, catapults, and comic books that filled the store's shelves. The decision to embrace the sport was simple: "Ralph Lauren owns tennis. So we decided to take table tennis." The company actually adopted a ping pong table when a friend of the designers couldn't fit it into their new apartment. (The table didn't actually fit in the Jack Spade office either, but they made room by getting rid of less important things like the conference table.) Special rules were developed to account for balls hitting the low light fixtures, and a handicap was given to the player on the west side of the room facing the afternoon sun. After the accounting department complained about the noise, the designers began to visit the few remaining table tennis clubs around the city; they soon figured that if they make bags to carry things, why not create one for their paddles and balls? The Jack Spade paddle case was born, in chocolate brown, khaki, black, and camouflage Waxwear, detailed with a fetching suit stripe lining.

Spade's ping pong design kick could not be shaken. Upon selling Jack Spade and establishing Partners & Spade, a storefront and studio off the Bowery in Manhattan, one of his first projects was a limited-edition ping pong sneaker in partnership with K-Swiss. To enter the store and see the simple yet elegant sneakers—individually numbered in a run of 266—lined up in museum-quality display cases is to finally see the sport on the pedestal it deserves. But Spade is not yet finished; his dream is to develop a customized line of ping pong equipment and distribute it nationwide. "If Nieman Marcus can sell a branded yacht in their catalogue, J.Crew should be selling their own table tennis bats. . . . I will not be happy until I have turned the sport into the Ultimate Fighting Championship for slackers."

Top left: Jack Spades groundbreaking wax paddle case. *Bottom left:* K-Swiss subtly stylish limited edition ping pong kicks.

Smash Hits!

Because there are few sounds more poetic and inspiring than the natural rhythm of the table tennis rally, ping pong and music have an inextricable emotional history of codependence. The "ping-pong" recording style frees the track to bounce (or ping pong) between speakers. Alvino Rey, father of the pedal steel, used his "famous Console Guitar" to record the definitive album *Ping Pong*. The front cover portrayed two busty beauties desperately using both fore- and backhand to fend off an orgy of ping pong balls as the liner notes proclaim "never did a gayer, brighter bunch of sounds get bounced around than these."

Enrique Iglesias sullied the game with his insipid 2007 single, "Do You Know (the Ping Pong Song)" His record company forced him to add the subtitle to help marketing and boost sales, tarnishing the reputation of our beloved sport and making us all feel used and dirty in the process. Israel's entry to the 2000 Eurovision Song Contest was a more worthy standard-bearer for the game. Ping Pong was a Tel Aviv quartet who courted controversy by unfurling Syrian flags as a finale to their act, scandalizing the Jewish state and forcing the Israeli television network to take the unprecedented step of disowning their own representatives. We tracked down band member Roy Arad, who revealed their motivation. "We thought ping pong games between China and the USA brought peace. It became a challenge, because I have a rare phobia surrounding ball games and cannot watch people play ping pong, soccer, or even *matka,* Israeli beach tennis. When we were in the band, everyone asked me to actually play ping pong. It was nightmare."

Our favorite track comes from Plastic Bertrand, Belgium's answer to Johnny Rotten, who followed up his rollicking 1977 global smash "Ça plane pour moi" with the single "Ping Pong," a piece of poetry that artfully compared a game of table tennis to the human emotion of love. Plastic reveals who he is in love with on the cover of the record; he is portrayed solo, enjoying a refreshing malt beverage after an arduous yet no doubt victorious stint at the table. Thankfully, his battery of sweatbands have done the job, and he is dry as a bone. If this book had a theme song, this would be it, yet when it was released in 1982, the song was ahead of its time. It flopped everywhere, charting only in Italy.

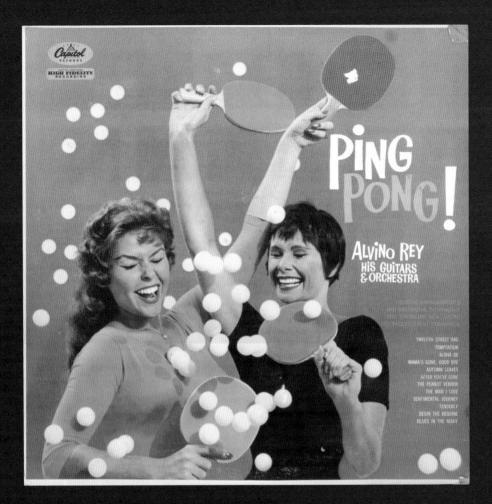

Album cover of *Ping Pong!* by Alvino Rey and His
Guitars & Orchestra, 1960.

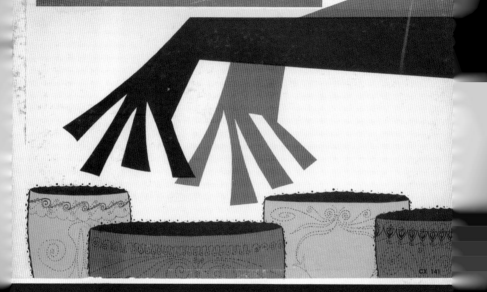

* FABULOUS *
PING***PONG
BONGO
PERCUSSION

CORONET RECORDS

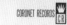

CX 141

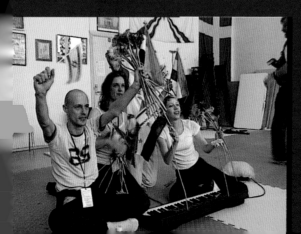

Top: Fabulous Ping Pong Bongo Percussion, Kaino and his African percussion group, circa 1955.

Opposite page: I Wants a Ping-Pong Man, A Coontown Determination by Howard Whitney, 1902.

Bottom: Israeli Eurovision provocateurs, Ping Pong, 2000.

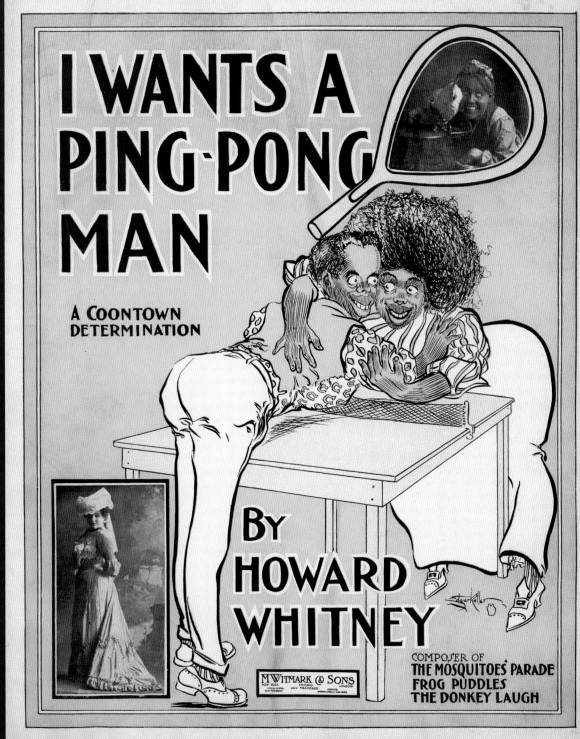

CHUCK SAGLE AND HIS ORCHESTRA

PING PONG PERCUSSION

PING PONG PERCUSSION

Who's Sorry Now
The Sheik of Araby
For Me and My Gal
How Come You Do Me Like You Do
My Honey's Lovin' Arms
When the Saints Go Marching In
Make Love to Me
Cuddle Up a Little Closer
Stars Fell on Alabama
Muskrat Ramble
Someday Sweetheart
High Society

Ping Pong Percussion by
Chuck Sagle and Orchestra,
circa 1950.

Ping Pong EP, SNFU, 2000.

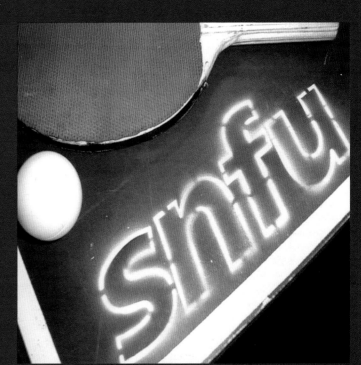

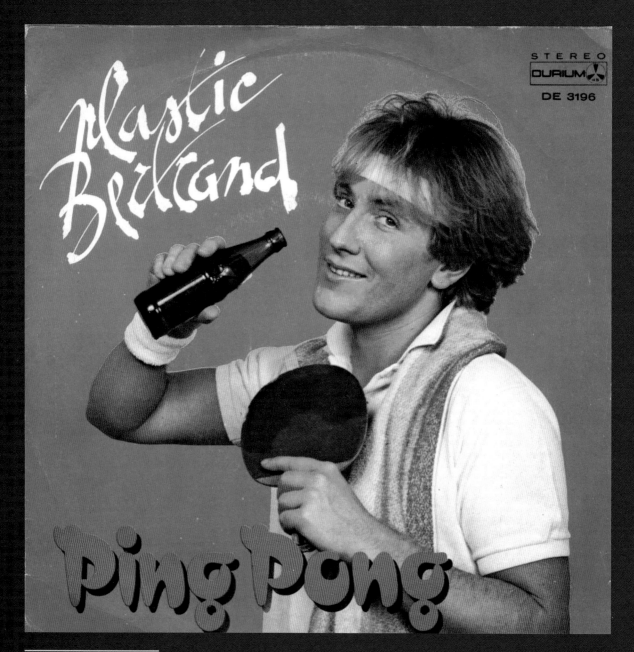

Ping Pong by Plastic
Bertrand, 1977.

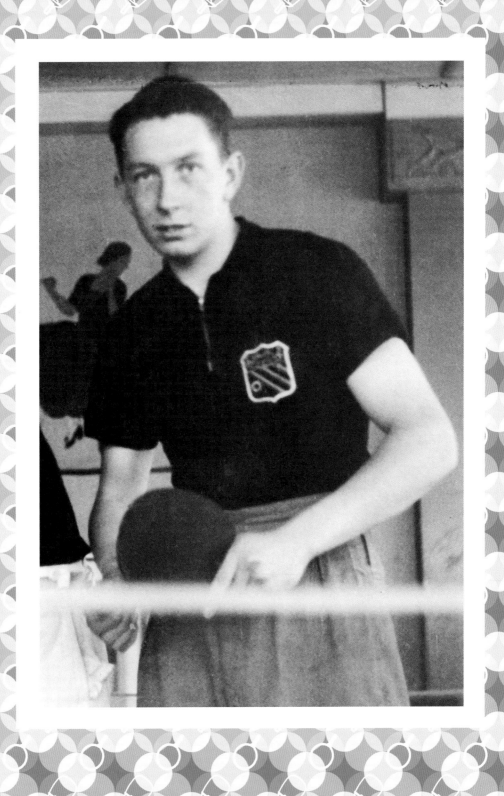

OUT OF FASHION

BY HARRY EVANS

They came out of prewar Eastern Europe with their magic names: Zolan Mechlovits, Miklos Szabados, Stanislav Kolar, Viktor Barna, Ivan Andreadis, Bohumil Vana, Richard Bergmann. . . . They were in their slim teens, mostly, when they showed the world how to play table tennis, the thrillingly classic game with hard-pimpled rubber before the spongers ruined it all. (The exception was 240 pounds of dancing dynamite called Ferenc Sido from Hungary.)

Physically, their movements resembled the cut and thrust of fencing—never having fought with a rapier, I'm quoting my ping pong friend B. Barry, who directs epic duels for the movies and the stage when not unleashing his own forehand drive: "The mental state and the skill are of equal measure. The happy result is death without blood." The names from Hungary, Austria, Yugoslavia, and Czechoslovakia were reminiscent of those attached to famous chess matches, and that's what they were psychically. The maneuvers around and beyond the table, probing for weaknesses in defense, were as intense in their concentration, and as inventive in combining elements: one thinks of the corner-to-corner topspin drives as if they were bishops striking along the diagonals, the angled push shots as acquisitive pawns.

I was eliminated by the French national champion in the early rounds of the English Open championships in 1948, but I was there with 5,000 others to see the epic contest between the two who'd made it to the men's singles final. Could the world's greatest attacking player penetrate the defenses of the world's greatest defender? The fleet-footed Czech Bohumil Vana, his hair held back by a dark headband, was so economical in every move he never gasped or smiled; he was, to borrow a phrase, a lean, mean fighting machine. He could drive a defender back and back with a fusillade of forehands all round the table. Bergmann by contrast seemed a plodder, squat and solid, lead against mercury, but he had a retrieving capacity the like of which was never equaled in hardbat play and the ferocity of a beast. Against Hungary's maddeningly consistent defender Ferenc Soos, he was two games down but provoked Soos to attack by lobbing high balls. Soos, in the end, could not resist the humiliation of failing to kill such easy returns, but he didn't have the equipment to put the ball where Bergmann couldn't reach it. He went down 13–21 to the man who became known as Richard the Lionheart, so often did he snatch victory from defeat; indeed, no other player in the game's history has ever matched his resilience.

On the night of the Vana-Bergmann encounter, the 5,000 in the great King's Hall at Belle Vue, Manchester, were tensely silent when they weren't stomping and cheering. Normally the crowd is with the adventurous attacker, but this night they were rooting for Bergmann, since he'd become a naturalized British citizen (and served in the Royal Air Force), and not since Fred Perry won the singles in 1929 had any other than the East Europeans won. (Perry retired to take up lawn tennis, because, he said, it was easier, and won three Wimbledons in a row.) The silence I've mentioned, as we held our breaths in the long rallies, was not complete. As the struggle between Vana and Bergmann developed, here was that marvelous sound lost to the sponge game of hardbat striking the ball, a crisp, rhythmic, hypnotizing sound that only looks ridiculous when rendered into words—plickety-plock-plick is one variation, kerplock-kerplock is another. The amplified dialogue of challenge and response made the match all the more comprehensible to the audience. The exchanges were fast, but it wasn't just a question of speed. There was the way the electrifying Vana angled Bergmann farther and farther away from the center, and then with an almost imperceptible body swivel switched sides, or hit down the center into Bergmann's gut, the Achilles heel of every player on the planet.

Except Bergmann. Wherever the ball was, Bergmann was sure to be, his footwork taking him into perfect position, often with his back to the barrier, giving wonder to the sea of spectators. Was this an illusion? Was it the blur of a man scooping the ball from twenty feet back the same man a moment later back at the center of the table picking up a delicate drop shot, responding with an angled push shot, and a short series of forehand drives? The drives were not as pretty as Vana's, more of a heaving effort than Vana's lethal silkiness, but they were consistent and effective. Bergmann lost the first game 17–21, romped home 21–10 in the second by blocking half-volleys that disturbed Vana's rhythm, and then it was a point-by-point struggle. Bergmann returned Vana's drives low over the net and deep into Vana's court, but he angled them wide, too. Vana was then tempted to run round to make his pet stroke, but the geometry reduced his strike area, leading him to hit off the table. I thought Bergmann deliberately returned some balls short so that Vana had an easy drop shot, but nothing was easy against Bergmann. He was ready, and time and time again his speed was able to transmute a seemingly "dead ball" into an opening for attack. He edged that third game 21–19, and in the fourth game a demoralized Vana went down 21–11 to make Bergmann the champion. I was hooked for life.

The domination of the East Europeans was really broken first in 1949 by that nineteen-year-old American kid, the Needle, as he was called on the Lower East Side, the graceful bespectacled joker, Marty

Reisman. In a five-set final, he beat the elegant Hungarian Victor Barna, five-time world champion, inventor of the backhand flick and one of the most gentlemanly players: when I played him years later, he forbore the humiliation he might easily have inflicted. Reisman is the only American male ever to have won the English Open, wowing Wembley Stadium's 10,000 spectators with a glimpse of what was then the fastest forehand kill in the world.

But that's not his greatest distinction. He is the real hero of table tennis because he has pretty well single-handedly kept the classic game alive to enjoy its present resurgence. Alone among the greats, he did not switch to sponge when it swept the world after the 1952 world championships in Bombay. Hiroji Satoh, an indifferent player in the classic game and only an alternate on the Japanese team, became world champion on the strength of his new secret weapon, resilient foam rubber that imparted unreadable spins. He baffled all the classic players with his soundless paddle silencer and "sling shot." Reisman tested his own skill in a return match in Osaka against Satoh that convulsed Japan. He stuck to his hard pimpled rubber panel and before an astounded capacity crowd beat Satoh fair and square.

Sponge should have been banned when it first infiltrated. It was like a boxer climbing into the ring with iron filings in his gloves. The president of the International Table Tennis Federation, the Honorable Ivor Montagu (who happened to be an eccentric English aristocrat and a Communist) thought sponge might be a great equalizer that would open the sport to novices. He prevailed: sponge was legalized, a decision that doomed us to fifty years of gimmickry. The effect was the opposite of Montagu's egalitarian intent. It closed off the sport.

Technology ran amok. About 900 bewildering varieties of sponge came into use. Players came to use different surfaces on forehand and backhand. The unknowable combination means that, irrespective of the opponent's skill and determination, you face a million variations of equipment—900 times 900 equals 810,000 possible mixes of backhand and forehand sponge. And on top of that there's this matter of glue; the substance holding the different material on backhand and forehand was also found to have an effect on spin and speed. Players started changing glue midmatch, cooking up their concoctions in a break. Tournaments smelt like a Formula One racetrack.

The lunacy took the fun out of playing and killed table tennis as a spectator sport. Sponge is unpredictable and very hard to control even after continuous training. The sponge players who followed Satoh are much better athletes, but the games they play have been generally unwatchable—basically trick serves accompanied by foot stamping (if the umpire doesn't object) and then a fast loop, which either wins or loses the point. The typical sponge point is won after only three or four exchanges, by contrast with ten, twenty, thirty, or forty in a classic game. The monotony of sponge matches—wham, bam, thank you ma'am—is the reason why, the Olympics apart, finals that once attracted thousands average only a handful of aficionados in the stands. And for the beginner, the trickiness of the sponge racket is the reason why table tennis has not until recently attracted and sustained the interest of millions of basement players, as it once did.

When sponge devastated the sport, I stopped playing regularly in the 1960s. In the mid-1970s, in the wake of the Cultural Revolution in China, the first sign of a thaw in Sino-American relations was of course the invitation of the American table tennis team to play in China. British-Chinese relations were not very good for a time. For some weird reason, staff at the China Office (it did not have embassy status) came out into the street and attacked a police cordon with axes and clubs. Taking a leaf out of Chou En-lai's book, I invited the Chinese to play a table tennis match against a team of five I would assemble at the *Sunday Times* I edited. I practiced with the unfamiliar sponge with the country star Alan Sherwood. On the night at the *Sunday Times* office, the newspaper team beat the diplomats. The Chinese asked for a return match. I didn't recognize anyone from the first encounter. They'd scoured Europe for a completely new team. It all came down to the last game of the night. I led 18–17 when my opponent had service. His first serve looked straightforward enough. My hit went off the side, 18–18. I put the second off the other side of the table, 18–19. I put the third in the net, 18–20, and the fourth off the table again. My opponent had saved up four freakish sponge services. By the time I'd just about worked out the convolutions of racket and posture producing the varied spins, it was too late. I'd lost the game 18–21 and the match 4–5.

I don't grumble at the result. The mysterious newcomer won fair and square by the terms of the sport then. I played a few more times with my new sponge racket and did all right with wristy backhands and fast sweeping forehands, but it wasn't half as much fun or half as satisfying. Then Reisman came into my life. I hadn't seen him at the English Open in 1949—I was in the Royal Air Force—but fifty years after his triumph I met him quite by chance in New York when he was celebrating his seventy-third birthday. "Why don't you start playing again?" he asked. I showed up at a city gym with the paddle I'd used against the Chinese, and he played with his Reisman paddle of hard pimpled rubber. Taking my punishment, as he switched from defense to attack, and hearing once again the sound of celluloid on hardbat, my imagination retrieved slow-motion images of those graceful East Europeans. I abandoned sponge.

The classic game would have been lost but for Reisman. "I was so disgusted with what had happened to its innocence, purity, and simplicity," he says. The icon kept the embers of the sport alive by a willingness to bet his last buck on himself in challenge matches—one for $10,000 against Jimmy Butler, forty-two years his junior. Watchers were mesmerized when they saw quicksilver Reisman—and heard his patter, for he's a showman, a wisecracking reciter of Shakespeare who likes to upend a slim cigarette on one end of the table and split it neatly in two with a ball from a precise forehand. In the 1960s and 1970s he ran a New York table tennis salon where the *Daily News* reported Bobby Fischer found relief from the rigors of chess. Dustin Hoffman, Kurt Vonnegut, and Matthew Broderick were regulars. Murray Kempton observed in 1971: "To come upon Reisman is like finding some perfect specimen of a classic age, thin as a blade, the step a matador's, the stroke a kitten's."

Players began to return to the classic game in the late 1970s. Local groups coalesced to form the USATT hardbat committee, led by Scott Gordon, a Sacramento computer scientist. In 1997, a national hardbat championship was staged. Reisman snatched the title, an athletic feat not thought possible for a sixty-seven-year-old who demolished the field in an open-age event and recaptured the USATT national title he had won thrity-eight years before. His inspired victory—he beat a semifinalist opponent 21–0 in one game—was a turning point, encouraging players frustrated by the sponge chaos. The insurrection the renegade Reisman started has continued to grow, a return to the classic game that has rejuvenated the sport in America and abroad. In an audacious attempt to resuscitate the bare bones of table tennis, at the age of seventy-nine, he has redesigned the simple sandpaper racket, one benign regression short of the original parchment and bare wood. "The sandpaper paddle," he says, "affords the purest reflection of a player's innate skills." The $100,000 hardbat championship in Las Vegas in 2009 was the brainchild of Reisman. As well as restoring the classic game, they're piquantly restoring the classic name; the sandpaper group is now planning the $200,000 Ping Pong World Championships.

Let the trophy cup for the winner be known hereafter as the Reisman: Bergmann was the world's greatest retriever, but Marty Reisman, the kid from the Lower East Side, has gone one better than Bergmann. He has saved the whole sport.

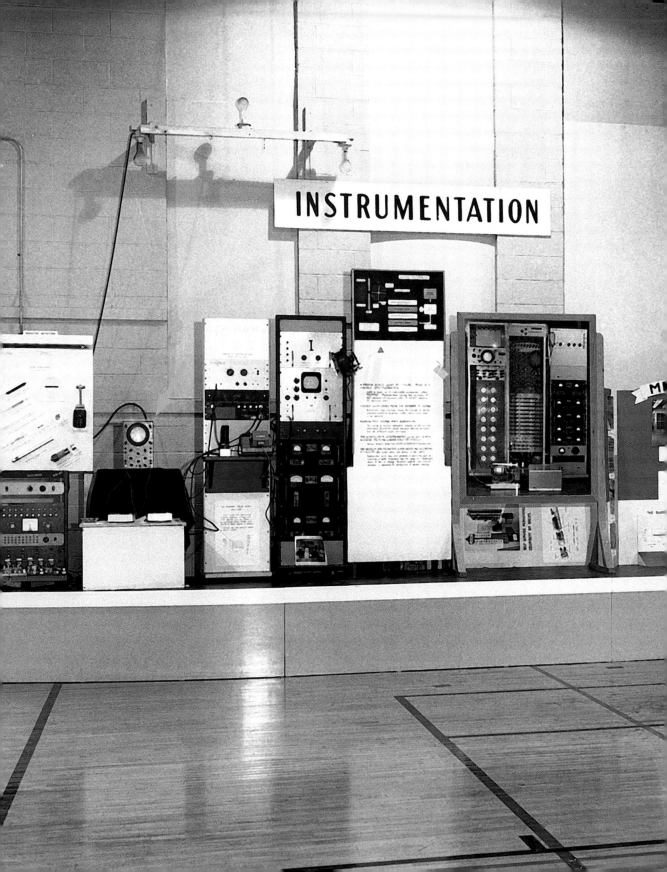

INSTRUMENTATION

AUGMENTED REALITY

WHEN PONG BECAME *PONG*, AND EVERYTHING AFTER

William Higinbotham began his career at Los Alamos, developing components for the first atomic bomb. He ended his career as a leader of the Federation of American Scientists, a group dedicated to combating nuclear proliferation. Somewhere in the middle (1958, specifically), he was just a staff scientist trying to liven up a boring vistors' day at the Brookhaven National Laboratory. Higinbotham decided to debut a recent project—an unlikely contraption combining an analog computer and an oscilloscope. The result was something entirely new—a game, displayed on a screen, that could be played by adjusting knobs and buttons. The game itself, however, was strangely familiar: a tiny ball bouncing back and forth over a low perpendicular barrier.

Unfortunately, Higinbotham made the mistake of naming this game "Tennis for Two." Tennis players, a stiff, fearful bunch, wouldn't come near the thing, and the game never left the confines of the lab. Higinbotham's contraption was dismantled two years later.

In the subsequent half century, Higinbotham's hobby has, of course, grown into one of this millennium's primary obsessions, particularly among the

Brookhaven National Laboratory, 1958. The arrow points to the groundbreaking oscilloscope.

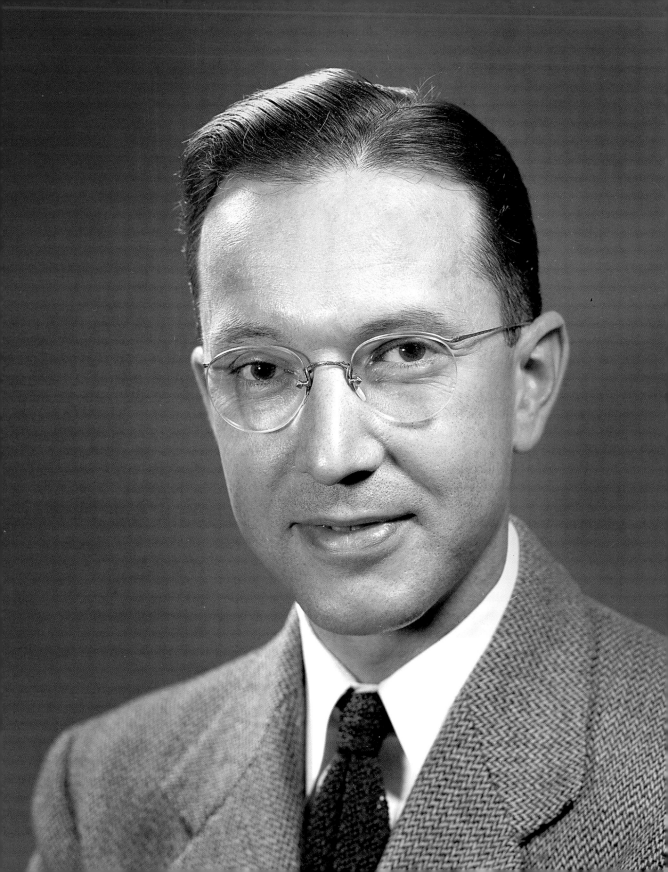

younger generation, those obese infants spreading their slimy trails across our civilization. Some people might see this as a bad sign for ping pong: another traditional pastime crowded out by the relentless march of technology. Some people, of course, are fools—for ping pong is both the origin and destination of video entertainment, the alpha and omega of this blip of beeps and boops. Truth is, video games are but yet another manifestation *of* ping pong, a medium with which to spread the joys thereof to a new century of limbless, spaceless, or friendless aficonados.

A few years after Higinbotham's overlooked invention, a group of young engineers at MIT made another attempt: Spacewar! [*exclamation theirs*]. The game was a significant technological breakthrough, but this fact was appreciated by early computer scientists and almost no one else. Next, Ralph Baer at the Magnavox labs developed a series of groundbreaking games for their Odyssey project: Fox & Hounds, Firefighter, and a "bucket-filling" challenge. It was a period of remarkable innovation, but the games were just not enough *fun*.

Then Baer hit upon his masterwork: "TV Ping-Pong," which built upon Higinbotham's early insight while avoiding his misguided title. Ping pong was a perfect platform for the limited power of the early computers: simple mathematical foundations leading to endless possibility and variation. The graphics were brutally simple—just one line per paddle, a dotted line for the net, and a square for the ball—but the gameplay was addictive. There was an intuitive purity to the physical parameters: all angles and velocity, no sci-fi mumbo jumbo.

Enter Nolan Bushnell, young founder of a new company named Atari. Bushnell's first game, 1971's Computer Space, had been a failure; for the casual gameplaying population, raised on the shiny lights and ringing bells of pinball, the arid landscape of extraterrestrial warfare proved to be too off-putting. Despite a futuristic, curvaceous console (depicted in ads being caressed by an equally curvaceous woman), the game was universally rejected by teenagers and barflies across the nation.

For its next effort, Atari wanted something familiar, approachable even on a glowing green screen. Says Bushnell: "To be successful, I had to come up

William Higinbotham, father of video games.

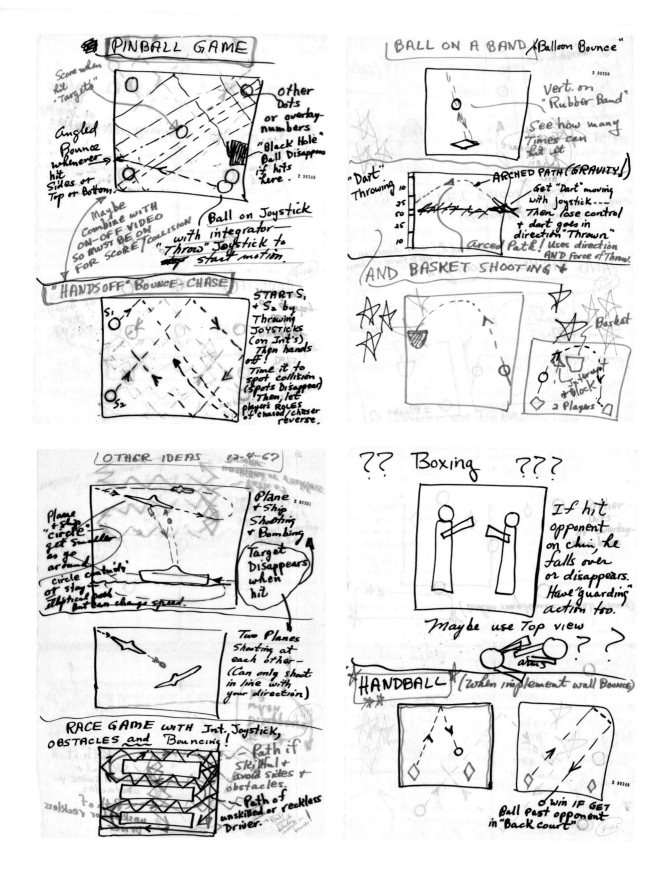

PINBALL GAME

Score when hit "Targets"

Other Dots or overlay numbers "Black Hole" Ball Disappears if hits here. 2 90348

Angled Bounce whenever hit Sides or Top or Bottom.

Maybe combine with ON-OFF VIDEO SO MUST BE ON FOR SCORE COLLISION

Ball on Joystick with integrator — "Throw" Joystick to start motion.

"HANDS OFF" BOUNCE - CHASE

S₁

S₂

STARTS₁ + S₂ by Throwing JOYSTICKS (on Int's) Then hands off! Time it to spot collision (Spots Disappear) Then, let player's ROLES of chased/chaser reverse.

BALL ON A BAND "Balloon Bounce"

2 90350

Vert. on "Rubber Band"

See how many Times can hit it

"Dart" Throwing

10
35
50
35
10

ARCHED PATH (GRAVITY!)

Get "Dart" moving with joystick --- Then lose control + dart goes in direction "Thrown"

Arced Path! Uses direction AND Force of Throw.

AND BASKET SHOOTING +

T

Basket

T

*Block

2 Players

OTHER IDEAS   02-4-67

Plane + Ship "circle" get smaller as go around — circle continuity or stay elliptical but can change speed.

Plane + Ship Shooting + Bombing

2 90351

Target Disappears when hit

Two Planes shooting at each other — (Can only shoot in line with your direction)

RACE GAME WITH Int. Joystick, OBSTACLES and Bouncing!

— Path if Skillful + avoid sides + obstacles.

— Path of unskilled or reckless Driver.

?? Boxing ???

If hit opponent on chin, he falls over or disappears. Have "guarding" action too.

Maybe use Top view

arms ? ?

HANDBALL (When implement wall Bounce)

T

2 90349

Win IF GET Ball past opponent in "Back court"

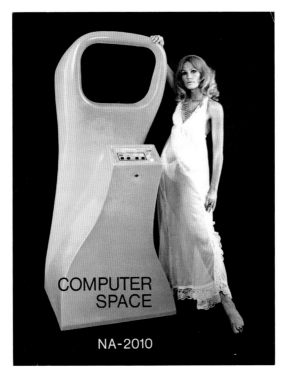

An ad for Atari's Computer Space, deemed less enticing than PONG, 1971.

with a game people already knew how to play, something so simple that any drunk in a bar could play." But not just *anything*; he didn't turn to billiards or darts or sexual harassment, other favored diversions of his desired demographic. No, only one pastime could really do the trick. Bushnell saw Baer's machine at the 1972 Magnavox Profit Caravan, and it confirmed his hunches. The name "Ping-Pong" was copyrighted by Parker Brothers, so they settled on PONG. The only instructions provided: "Avoid missing ball for high score"— nothing more was needed, so beloved and ingrained were the contours of the gameplay. (These principles were later distilled into the Nolan's Theorem, still a guiding force for programers and designers: "All the best games are easy to learn and difficult to master.")[1]

At the core of Bushnell's genius was a fact already known to half the world's population: there is no other form of live-action, head-to-head competition

1. This was followed by Albaugh's Corollary (named after a Mike Albaugh, an early Atari programmer): "The best games can be played with one hand, so you can have your beer or your girlfriend in the other."

Sketches by Bill Rusch of Magnavox, evaluating lesser, non-pong-based options, 1967.

that is more economically intuitive, equitable, and efficient with regards to space, time, and order than ping pong. Basketball requires high-tops and a ten-foot rim; football needs a hundred yards of grass and twenty additional participants; fencing asks grown men to wear a ponytail and a codpiece. Ping pong demands little more than three deflecting surfaces (two bats, a table) and a vector of pure physics (the ball)—while also sparing you the indignity of being crotch-poked by a Frenchman. The bouncing ball, the plain surface, the intuitive symmetry of incident angles: these are the baby building blocks of Newton's Second Law, the pure forces we gum with toothless comprehension even before ever picking up a paddle. PONG took the fundamental physics of ping pong (which in turn encapsulates the fundamental mechanics of competitive gameplay) and translated them into their simplest digital, monochromatic form—into the fundamentals of fun.

PONG was an instant sensation, leading to countless spinoffs and knock-offs: Rally, Paddleball, Winner, Quadrapong, Puppypong. (One classic variant was Breakout, created when Atari hired two young programers, Steve Jobs and Steve Wozniak, just a year before they founded their own company, Apple.) Each game had its own innovations, but they all shared the same inexhaustible core: a bouncing ball, a sliding paddle, a hated opponent. That last factor, the opponent, was another important development in the gaming world. At the time, the industry was dominated by pinball, an essentially solitary activity. PONG allowed for direct interaction, simultaneous competition—a social entry for maladjusted teens. Thus, video games began as a social phenomenon, a tavern icebreaker, a cross-cultural uniter for a nation torn asunder by the Vietnam War, Watergate, and the premiere of *Sanford and Son*.[2]

This golden age didn't last long. Video games soon lost their way. The refined minimalism of PONG was submerged in elaborate cartoony diversions: Pac-Man, then Mario, then Zelda—candy-colored obsessions for latchkey kids. Then, as these undersocialized youths grew up, a violent pseudorealism took the fore, with first-person shooters like Doom and Halo. The utopian

2. When asked his favorite video game, notable uniter Barack Obama said, "PONG . . . I loved that game."

224

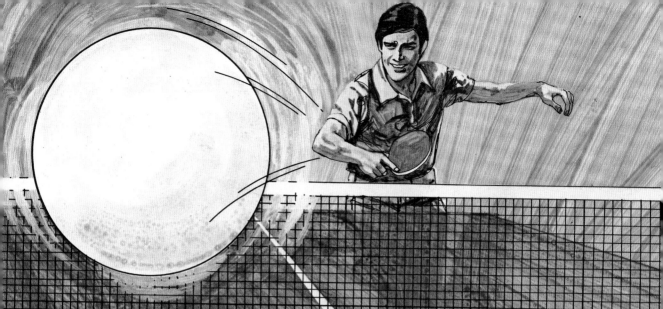

MIDWAY'S
TABLE-TENNIS

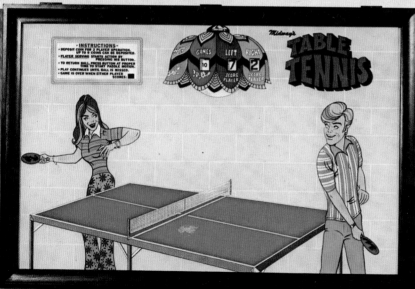

- 2-Player Competition
- Ball Speed determined by Player's S
- Wall mount or Pedestal mount availa
- Electronically or Mechanically played
- Dimensions: 46″ wide x 30″ high x 6″ d

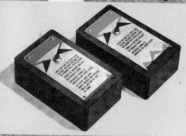

MM — MIDWAY MFG. CO. — 3750 River Road–Schiller Park, Illinois 60176   phone: (312) 678-1350

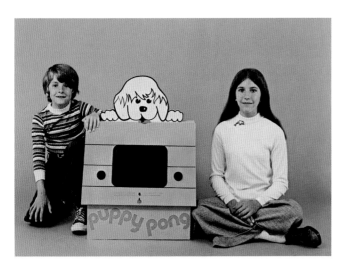

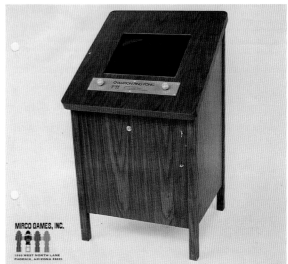

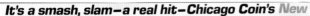

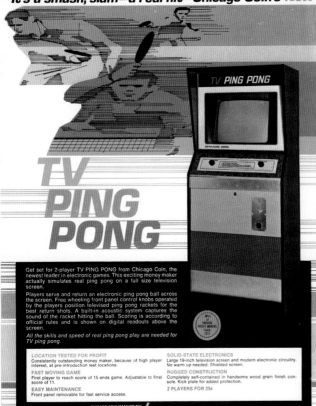
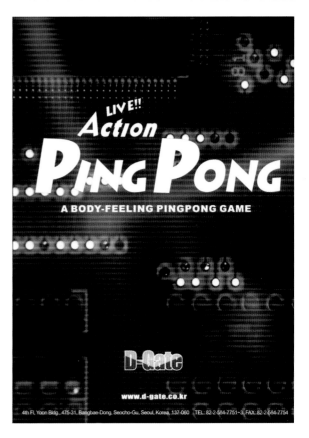

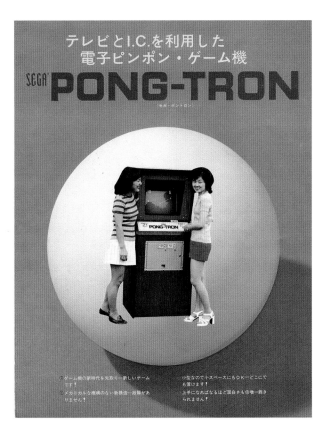

テレビとI.C.を利用した
電子ピンポン・ゲーム機

SEGA PONG-TRON

(セガ・ポントロン)

- ゲーム機の新時代を先取り一新しいゲームです！
- メカニカルな機構のない新構造一故障がありません！
- 小型なので小スペースにもOK—どこでも置けます！
- 上手になればなるほど面白さも倍増一飽きられません！

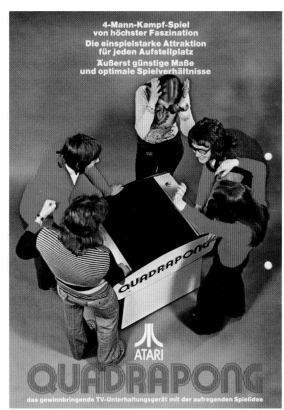

4-Mann-Kampf-Spiel
von höchster Faszination
Die einspielstarke Attraktion
für jeden Aufstellplatz
Äußerst günstige Maße
und optimale Spielverhältnisse

ATARI

QUADRAPONG

das gewinnbringende TV-Unterhaltungsgerät mit der aufregenden Spielidee

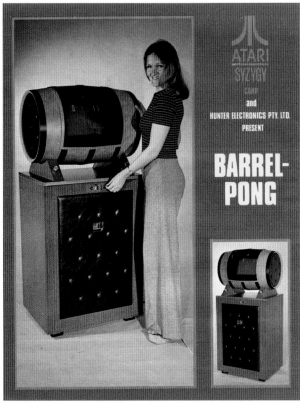

ATARI SYZYGY CORP
and
HUNTER ELECTRONICS PTY. LTD.
PRESENT

BARREL-PONG

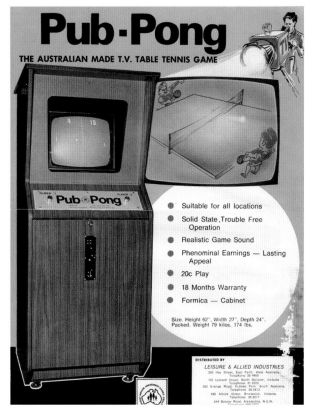

Pub·Pong

THE AUSTRALIAN MADE T.V. TABLE TENNIS GAME

- Suitable for all locations
- Solid State, Trouble Free Operation
- Realistic Game Sound
- Phenominal Earnings — Lasting Appeal
- 20c Play
- 18 Months Warranty
- Formica — Cabinet

Size. Height 62", Width 27", Depth 24".
Packed. Weight 79 kilos, 174 lbs.

promise of PONG had devolved into solipsistic masturbation occasionally interrupted by high-school massacres. And ping pong itself wasn't doing too great, either.

But it is always darkest before the dawn. The first signs of hope came when Rockstar Games, developers of Grand Theft Auto—one of the more unPONG-like games ever made—unveiled their eagerly anticipated follow-up: Table Tennis. The game was a hyperreal depiction of just that—two players across a table, no weak storyline or adjustable outfits, just the game itself. Building on three decades of computing advances, riffing not on PONG but the ur-text itself, Rockstar's creation was a bold return to core values—gameplay values, entertainment values, human values: a bouncing ball, a hated opponent. Ping pong was no longer just a platform, a familiar vehicle; it had become a destination, an ideal of fun to be asymptotically pursued by a new generation of game designers. Video games were coming home.

This journey took another step forward with the introduction of the Wii in 2006; two of the nine minigames from Nintendo's *Wii Play* were ping pong derivatives. The first was Laser Hockey, a misleadingly named update of PONG, pharmacologically amplified with increased velocity, an angled paddle, and neon colors. The second, Table Tennis, was merely ping pong *reductio ad awesomnum*. The "players" (just disembodied hands and paddles, really) were controlled via flicks of the wrist, with no intermediating buttons or joysticks needed. The goal was now the *physical experience* of actually playing ping pong: the stabs, the spins, the slams. We're not there yet, of course. But the advances of this millennium are certainly encouraging.

The most exciting gaming advances of the twenty-first century, however, are not taking place on the console but rather in the laboratory. Florian Mueller and Martin Gibbs at the University of Melbourne have invented a three-player ping pong game, played over long-distance networks against video-projected opponents but nevertheless using real paddles and balls. Mueller and Gibbs' initial goal was to explore how our bodies interact with technology, and how this can produce deeper social activity; the question was what sport to use as a platform for this investigation. "We tried soccer, but it became

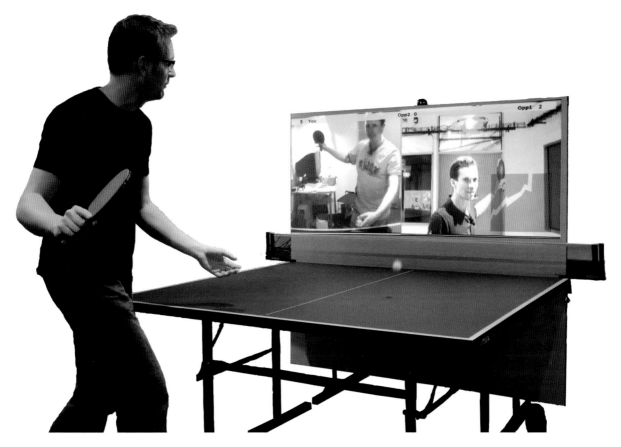

Mueller and Gibbs's three-way long-distance ping pong in action.

very competitive," says Mueller. "People wanted to hurt each other." Ping pong soon stepped forward as an ideal blend of battle and brotherhood, competition and conversation.

Rather than the typical holy grail of virtual reality, the aim here is *augmented* reality. As Mueller puts it, "Our goal was not to simulate table tennis. Our goal was to learn from it." The players hold real bats, hitting real balls, trying to defeat a real opponent; that opponent, however, is across town or across the continent. Much like Baer and Bushnell thirty years earlier, Mueller and Gibbs have utilized ping pong as a platform to explore new forms of gameplay and interaction. And this quest is still in its infancy. "Ideally we could scale it further, to a hundred tables or a thousand tables," explains Mueller. "I think it would be fantastic to have a table tennis competion in which dozens and dozens or hundreds and hundreds of players compete against each other all at once"—a battle royale of international fellowship.

While Mueller and Gibbs are interested in integrating physical activity into the human-computer gaming interface, Rainer Goebel at Maastricht University is attempting just the opposite: eliminating the need for even a joystick, replacing it with pure *mind control*. At this point, it seems hardly necessary to mention that his vehicle for these experiments is a game known as "brain pong." Two competitors sit within fMRI machines; by controlling their own brain waves, they are able to move a virtual paddle and bounce a ball toward their opponent. Goebel is unconcerned with the social factors that attracted Mueller and Gibbs; his goal is immediate comprehension, a purest form of gameplay. Ping pong turns out to be equally suited for both these realms; the disparate purposes are united in the shared human hunger for fun.

Throughout labs, arcades, and basements around the world, ping pong serves as an enduring metric for gaming's technological progress and a bell-wether for the underlying dreams and fears of a culture—whether a yearning for physical connection across distances, or a mistrust of our own bodies. To comparatively pong across the generations of gaming platforms—from Higinbotham's flickering oscilloscope to Rockstar's *Table Tennis* on today's hi-def consoles, and onto untold experimental mechanisms—is to press one's tongue against the cross-sectional glacier sampling tube that tells us precisely how each successive generation has sought to re-create essential *fun* in a collection of bytes and pixels.

A skeptic might ask: *why*? Why go to all this trouble to simulate the thrills of ping pong, when the real thing is right here? I have wondered this myself, I must admit. But the future is a long time, and we need to be prepared for the strange worlds to come. Imagine, perhaps, an environmentally ravaged landscape with no wood to build a table. Or an overpopulated urban sprawl without *room* for a table. Or a violent and/or disease-ridden dystopia in which we cannot leave our dorm-cells but still crave a bit of healthy competition. Or

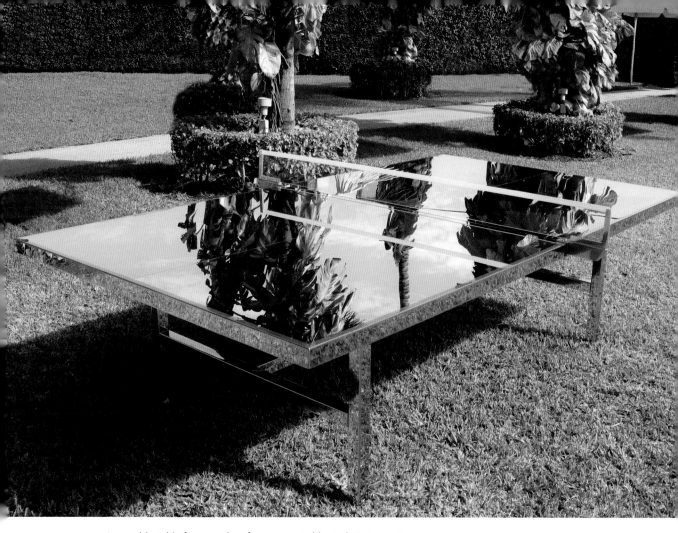

A possible table for a treeless future, created by Rirkrit Tiravanija.

even a distant descendent of current humans, evolved for a postindustrial civilization, with enormous postdiabetic livers but no opposable thumbs. The heroic programers of today are protecting ping pong for tomorrow's uncertain challenges. They understand their duty as stewards of our culture's most precious creations. Ping pong begat PONG, PONG begat a thousand offspring, and now those children are coming home.

A Century of Invention

Technological advancements in the ping pong realm aren't limited to the basement console or virtual-reality chamber; the game itself is a constant hotbed of innovation. And the midcentury game-changing debut of the sponge bat is just the metaphorical tip of the proverbial iceberg. A cruise through the United States Patent Office reveals a hundred years of imagination and struggle—the blank canvas whereupon the dreams of these lonely inventors are projected. Does the fact that these creations haven't appeared on the shelves of Toys "R" Us lessen their majesty? Just the opposite: the yearning for perfection and beyond is as old as the first caveman who realized a pointy rock might also be used as a good skull-basher.

This quest has lead to thousands of patents over the past century. There has been much tinkering with the paddle, some mild tinkering with the ball, and some extremely boring tinkering with the net clamps. But the real playground is the table: three-way, hourglass-shaped, corner-fitting, glass-enclosed . . . on and on, boldly anticipating the interior design challenges of a new millennium.

The text of the applications tends toward the mind numbing, with brief glimpses of the heroic madmen behind the creations. James Robert Harrell, for example, inventor of the circular rotating table (Patent #6,007,438), writes of a competitor: "Setting up this game would be more challenging than actually playing it." Zing! Nevertheless, the real glory of these trailblazers emerges in the diagrams and blueprints, multiangled and highly detailed visions of the world to come. Gaze upon them and tremble—what might have been, what still could be.

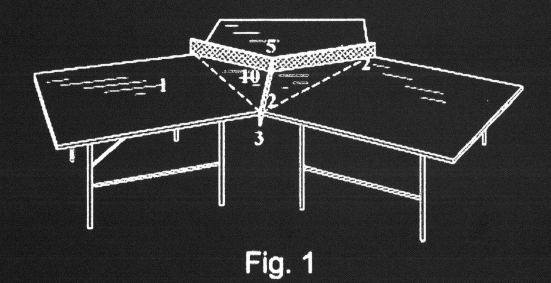

Fig. 1

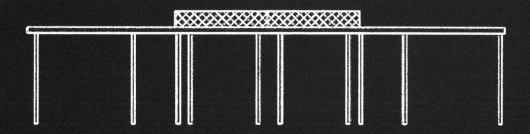

Fig. 2

#7,367,907. Inventors:
William M. Sutton and
Thomas Martinez.

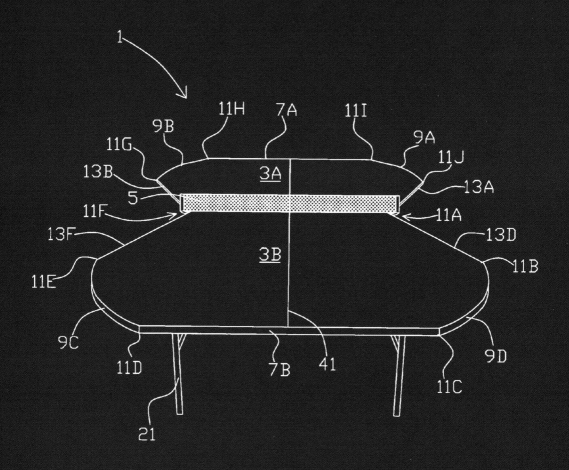

Above: #7,214,149. Inventors: Eric Nowitzky, Alfred Wright, and James Boyette. *Right:* #4,772,018. Inventor: Ronnie R. Inniger.

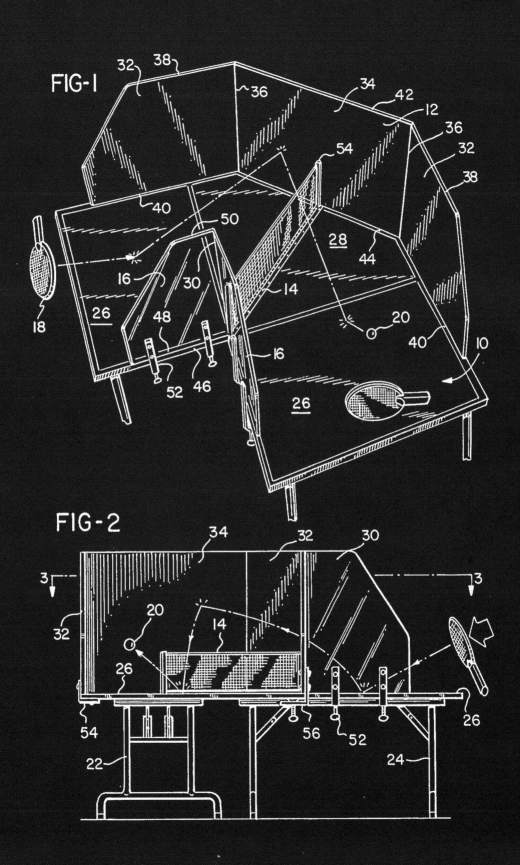

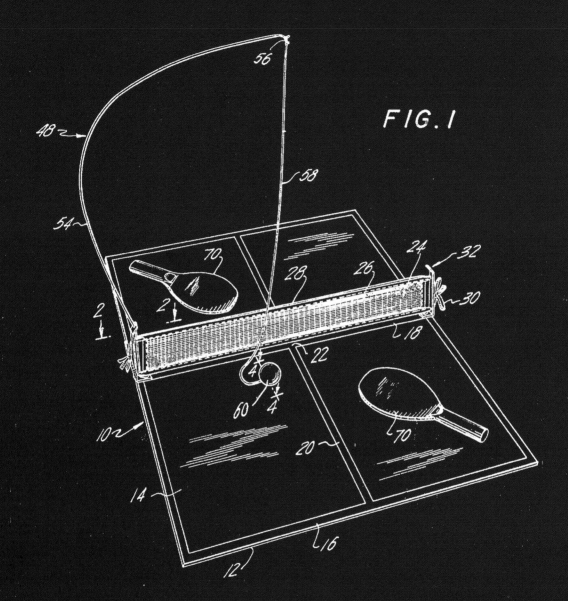

FIG. 1

#3,477,717. Inventor:
Theodore V. Clark.

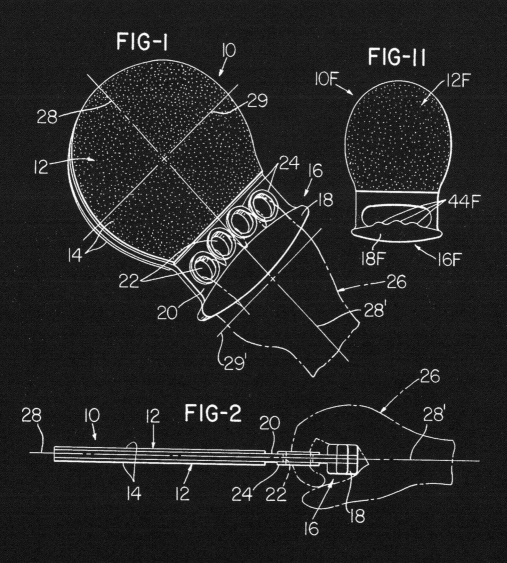

FIG-1

FIG-11

FIG-2

#3,674,268. Inventor:
Kenneth S. Shellman, Sr.

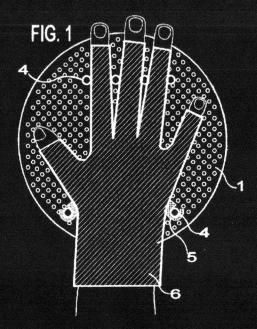

FIG. 1

FIG. 2

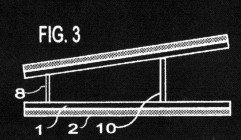

FIG. 3

FIG. 5

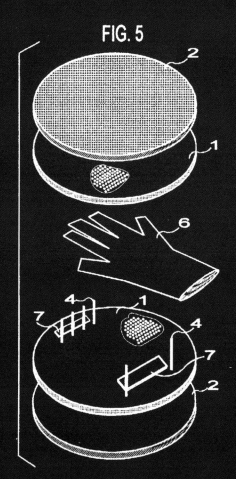

FIG. 4

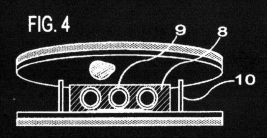

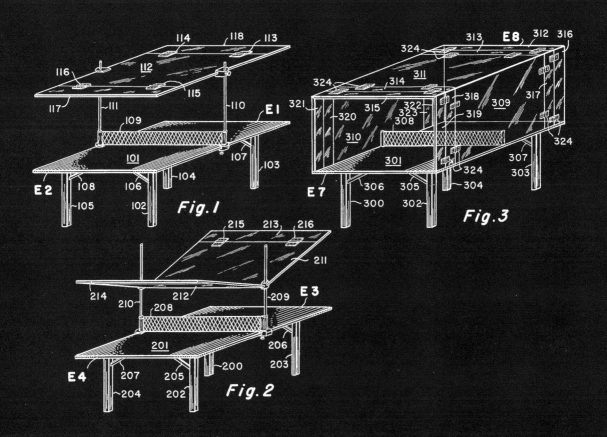

Left: #6,234,919. Inventors: Marion and Martin Mizerachi.
Above: #4,030,734. Inventor: Nicholas T. Castellucci.

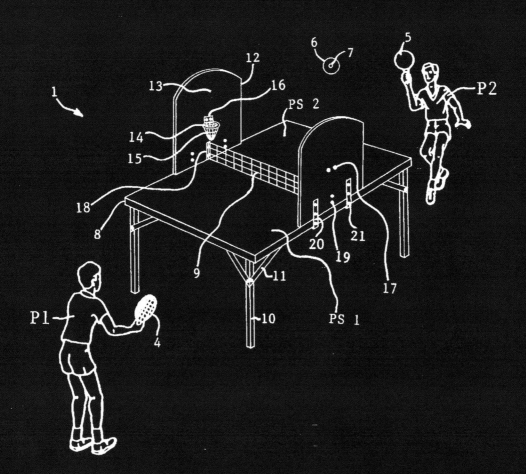

#5,655,979. Inventor: John
D. Blue.

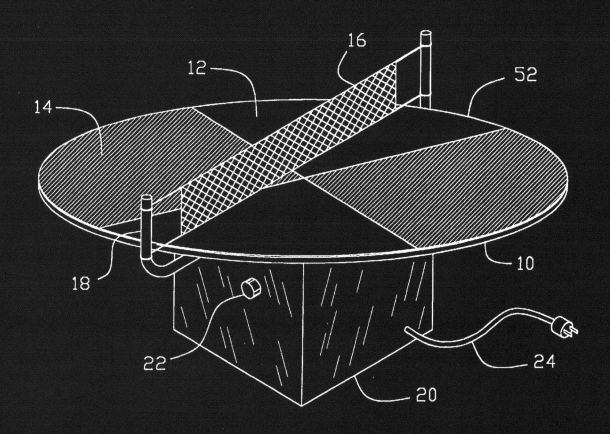

#6,007,438. Inventor: James
Harrell.

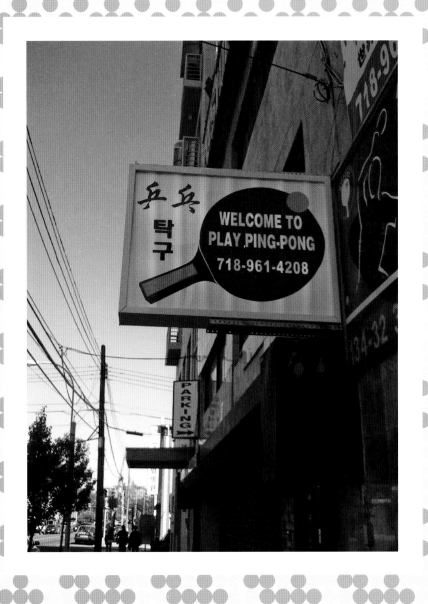

MY QUEST
BY WILL SHORTZ

As the crossword editor of the *New York Times*, I travel a lot for speaking engagements, puzzlers' conventions, and other reasons. As a table tennis enthusiast, I try to play at local table tennis clubs wherever I go.

At first, when I started visiting clubs, my goal wasn't to set a record. I just wanted to see how different clubs operated, to meet interesting people, to practice against different styles of play, and to stay in shape while I was on the road. But then it became an obsession to play at more U.S. clubs—and in more U.S. states—than anyone else in history.

As of March 2010, I've played at ninety-two clubs in twenty-two states. This is out of the 600 to 750 table tennis clubs that I estimate exist in the U.S., counting those affiliated with the USATT and National Collegiate Table Tennis Association, or legitimate clubs unaffiliated with anyone. I believe I already hold the record for U.S. clubs. But I don't intend to rest on my laurels. I'm always planning new trips.

As for when I'll be sure I have the record . . . there's probably no way ever to be sure. So, I'm just going to declare I have the record already. And if anyone wants to challenge me, I say—make your list of clubs with dates, as I've done, and we'll compare.

This map shows where and when I've played so far and my memories of some of these places.

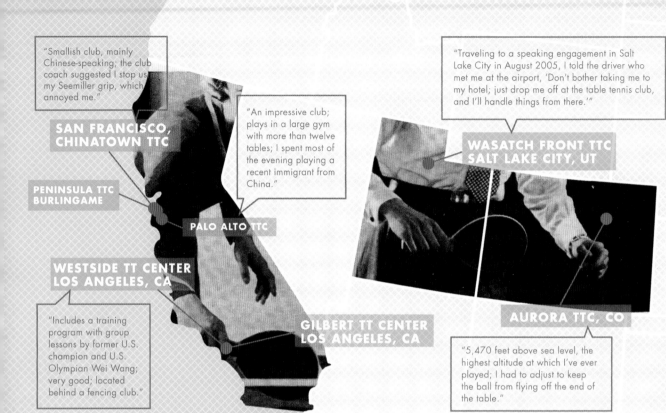

"Smallish club, mainly Chinese-speaking; the club coach suggested I stop using my Seemiller grip, which annoyed me."

SAN FRANCISCO, CHINATOWN TTC

PENINSULA TTC BURLINGAME

"An impressive club; plays in a large gym with more than twelve tables; I spent most of the evening playing a recent immigrant from China."

PALO ALTO TTC

"Traveling to a speaking engagement in Salt Lake City in August 2005, I told the driver who met me at the airport, 'Don't bother taking me to my hotel; just drop me off at the table tennis club, and I'll handle things from there.'"

WASATCH FRONT TTC SALT LAKE CITY, UT

WESTSIDE TT CENTER LOS ANGELES, CA

"Includes a training program with group lessons by former U.S. champion and U.S. Olympian Wei Wang; very good; located behind a fencing club."

GILBERT TT CENTER LOS ANGELES, CA

AURORA TTC, CO

"5,470 feet above sea level, the highest altitude at which I've ever played; I had to adjust to keep the ball from flying off the end of the table."

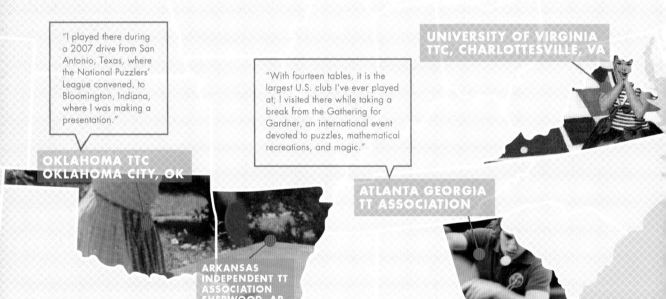

"I played there during a 2007 drive from San Antonio, Texas, where the National Puzzlers' League convened, to Bloomington, Indiana, where I was making a presentation."

"With fourteen tables, it is the largest U.S. club I've ever played at; I visited there while taking a break from the Gathering for Gardner, an international event devoted to puzzles, mathematical recreations, and magic."

UNIVERSITY OF VIRGINIA TTC, CHARLOTTESVILLE, VA

OKLAHOMA TTC OKLAHOMA CITY, OK

ATLANTA GEORGIA TT ASSOCIATION

ARKANSAS INDEPENDENT TT ASSOCIATION SHERWOOD, AR

"Just outside Little Rock; I played there after making a presentation on crosswords at the Clinton Presidential Library."

"In a handsome facility similar to the one in Glenview."

SCHAUMBERG TTC

"In a gorgeous community center, with a shower room, where I washed up before going out to dinner; loved it."

CHICAGO TTC GLENVIEW, IL

"Directed by five-time U.S. TT champion Danny Seemiller, with whom I played a match; let's just say he's a lot better than me."

SOUTH BEND TTC

"The director, Vincent Turner, held the club open late for me one evening in September 2007 so I could play after a speaking event."

CLEVELAND TT ASSOCATION

THREE RIVERS TT CENTER FORT WAYNE, IN

"Four tables; packed on the Saturday I was there."

CHICAGO SLAM TTC

KILLERSPIN TTC CHICAGO

AKRON TTC

"Where I got to participate in an intraclub tournament, with a pizza party, on the night I attended; very friendly."

KOKOMO TTC

CANTON TTC

"Largely Chinese; a mirror running the full length of the room made it impossible not to watch oneself play."

PURDUE UNIVERSITY TTC WEST LAFAYETTE

"The first stop on a fall 2009 table tennis road trip through the Midwest with my friend Robert Roberts (USATT-rated about 2570), during which we played at nine clubs over seven days; a complete blast."

XILIN TTC NAPERVILLE, IL

COLUMBUS TTC

INDIANA UNIVERSITY TTC BLOOMINGTON, IN

"In a very large space in a suburban shopping center with twelve tables; open seven nights a week; very nice."

"At my alma mater, the night before I delivered the 2008 commencement address; just what I needed to relax."

TABLE TENNIS CLUB OF INDIANAPOLIS

MONON CENTER TTC CARMEL, IN

"Whenever I think of starting my own club in New York, this is the one I imagine patterning it after; seven tables perfectly laid out in a long building, with a good floor and excellent lighting."

SOUTHERN INDIANA TT ASSOCIATION NEW ALBANY, IN

"Gorgeous community facility covering many sports, including volleyball and coed dodgeball, which I didn't play."

"The country's oldest TT club playing at the same location since 1935; after playing, about a dozen of us went out for pizza and beer."

One man, 71 cities, 82 clubs.

BINGHAMTON UNIVERSITY TT CLUB BINGHAMTON, NY

CHAMPLAIN VALLEY TTC BURLINGTON, VT

"Open seven days a week, dedicated to TT, with many good players; this is my favorite place to play in Boston."

"Visited during a three-day trip through the Northeast in spring 2009, while conducting crossword tournaments at Ivy League schools."

ACADEMY OF TT NEWTON, MA

WALTHAM TTC

BOSTON TT CENTER MEDFORD, MA

"On the upper floor of an old chicken house, with an outdoor barbecue on the day I was there; very enjoyable."

NASHUA TTC

NORTHEASTERN UNIVERSITY TTC BOSTON, MA

BAY STATE TTC SPRINGFIELD, MA

CHICKEN HOUSE TTC GORDONVILLE, PA

NANTICOKE TT, INC.

"Perhaps the most unusual club I've ever played at, built beneath the owner's suburban Long Island home; an amazing video at www.entt.org shows how it was done."

TUFTS TTC

"Where I played in a tournament in 2008, winning the U-1800 event."

GREATER BUFFALO TTC TONAWANDA, NY

FAIRFIELD TTC

RHODE ISLAND TT ASSOCIATION MANVILLE, RI

LANCASTER TTC

NEWTON TTC

EAST NORTHPORT TTC

GREATER HARTFORD TTC

LOWER NAUGATUCK VALLEY TT CENTER SHELTON, CT

MANOR TTC LANCASTER, PA

BOHEMIA TTC

CARLISLE AREA TTC CARLISLE, PA

"Two tables in the basement of owner Eleanor Leonhardt's house, with sofas at the side and a small table tennis museum at the end; I had a great evening here."

BALTIMORE TTC RANDALLSTOWN, MD

"Has two tables, one for better players, the other for less expert."

NEWARK TTC

ALLENTOWN/LEHIGH VALLEY TTC ALLENTOWN, PA

"In a gym at the University of Delaware."

POTTSGROVE TTC POTTSTOWN, PA

"I first visited there on a 2001 after-Christmas drive from Indiana, where I was visiting family, back home to New York, and I've returned several times since."

WESTERN MARYLAND TTC CUMBERLAND, MD

POTOMAC COUNTY TTC CABIN JOHN, MD

"Run by Jim Williams, known locally as 'Mr. Table Tennis', who's been playing for more than sixty years."

CLUB JOOLA ROCKVILLE, MD

"A stop-off on my way by car to a speaking engagement in White Sulphur Springs, W. Va."

"Has highly ranked coaches Jack Huang and Cheng Yinghua; I took a lesson from Cheng."

MARYLAND TT CENTER GAITHERSBURG, MD

"Has free monthly tournaments on Friday nights; the event is double elimination, so you keep playing until you lose twice; low-key with a friendly atmosphere."

"At a sports club."

MID HUDSON VALLEY TTC KINGSTON, NY

"Just two tables, but has good players, so it's worth a visit."

"Located at three different community centers; my home club since 2001, and still my favorite place to play."

RIVERTOWNS TTC HASTINGS, ARDSLEY, AND TARRYTOWN

"A gym at the Burke Rehabilitation Center; my second-most-played-at club."

"Marty Reisman's; my regular club in the late 1970s/early 1980s; Marty Reisman once played me with a chair instead of a paddle; I had to spot him fifteen points in a twenty-one-point gam . . . and he won."

BURKE TTC WHITE PLAINS, NY

PASSAIC TTC

FAIRLAWN TTC

"Cramped for space; has excellent coaching, though."

WEST SIDE TTC NEW YORK CITY

"Has one of the best coaches in the country, two-time World Seniors champion Yu Xiang Li; the first time I took a lesson from him, I went home with a list of eleven new things I'd learned."

MANHATTAN TTC NEW YORK CITY

WANG CHEN'S TTC NEW YORK CITY

"The club is so popular that the organizers restrict membership; usually they don't allow visitors, but they made an exception for me."

SPIN NEW YORK

NEW YORK INTERNATIONAL TTC FLUSHING, QUEENS

"A combination TT club/bar/restaurant/nightclub, opened in 2009; a new concept in table tennis, and very cool."

NEW YORK TTC FLUSHING, QUEENS

NEW YORK TT, INC. FLUSHING, QUEENS

MONROE TTC MONROE TOWNSHIP, NJ

FRIENDSHIP TTC FLUSHING, QUEENS

HOBOKEN TTC

BIG APPLE TTC ASTORIA, QUEENS

"One of the best clubs I've played at; dedicated to TT, open seven days a week; conducts monthly tournaments."

NEW YORK TT FEDERATION CHINATOWN, NEW YORK CITY

LOST BATTALION HALL TTC REGO PARK, QUEENS

NEW JERSEY TTC WESTFIELD, NJ

DYNAMO TTC BROOKLYN

CRANFORD TTC

"My home club during the mid 1980s; you need a New York City Parks and Recreation card to enter the building, but I recently talked my way in without one."

"Four tables in a parish community room."

"Mainly Russian; I've never met too many people named Alexei and played . . ."

"Lots of good players; I've visited twice, both times in the summer."

BROOKLYN NISON'S TT SCHOOL

PRINCETON UNIVERSITY TTC PRINCETON, NJ

WE CHALLENGE YOU TO A BEST OF THREE

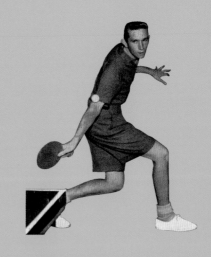

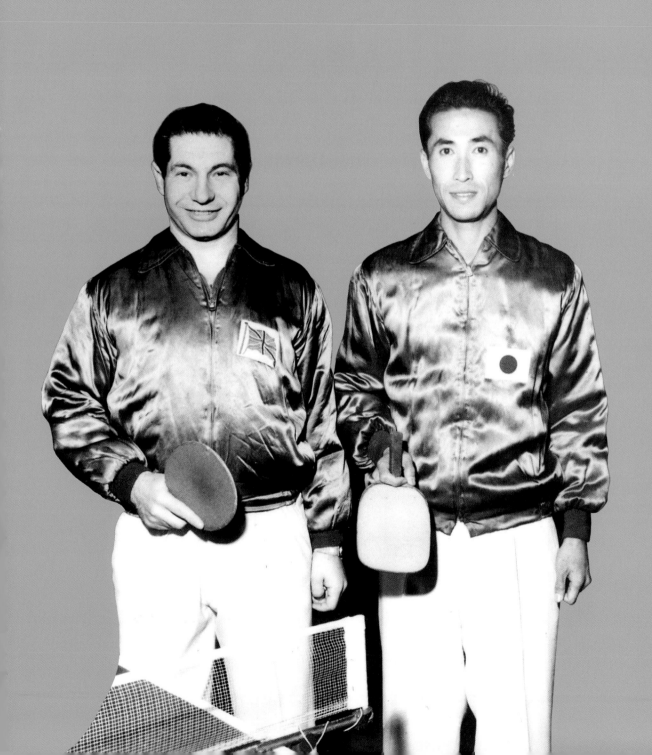

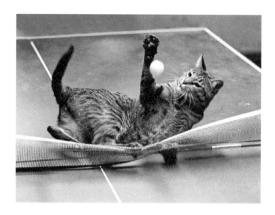

ACKNOWLEDGMENTS

It takes a special group of people to withstand the force of our bold truths. This book could not have come into existence without these loyal warriors.

Roger Bennett and Eli Horowitz thank the following:
Kate Lee of ICM, our first believer, along with the meticulous Larissa Silva; Carrie Kania, a visionary; Kate Hamill, a savvy and meticulous editor who wrangled our unruly romps; Jeremy Cesarec, Kevin Callahan, and Michael Barrs for their marketing genius; Cal Morgan and Mauro DiPreta for their golden touches throughout; Jayme Yen, our designer—inspired and patient in equal measure, you made it all pretty and clean; Chuck Hoey of the ITTF, an invaluable resource across the sea; and all photographers and collectors, including Malcolm Anderson, Eddy Portnoy, Ben Clarke, Albert Augustin, Niklas Nenzén, Anne Gunnison, Stas Kulesh, and Sean Hawkey.

Roger Bennett:
The game of ping pong and its lesser sister, tennis, were my life as a kid. Hitting the ball with menace and purpose gave me a real sense of confidence and accomplishment. Many of my happiest memories are of chop backhands and stinging forehand drives executed at my best friend Amanda Epstein's house. Her father was such a ping pong enthusiast, he purposely built a bungalow behind the family home to house his table. We would watch with wonder as he chiseled epically against my father, soaking up the power of my dad's high octane game. When I was eleven, I reached the final of my local club tournament, matched up against a player I knew I could crush. Needless to say, the crowd and the pressure got to me. I choked, and once I had flaccidly deposited the ball in the net on match point, I reacted in the manner television had deemed inappropriate to that time and place. Like John McEnroe, I was in tears, smashed my racquet, refused to shake my

victorious opponent's hand. My behavior was as violent as my parents were mortified. I have never played again.

My collection grew out of that moment of loss. Building it with Eli Horowitz has been a scholarly pursuit and a joy. Mr. and Mrs. Horowitz, your son is one of the most delightful persons I have encountered. Eli, thanks for your intellect, humor, patience, and friendship over the past four years of late-night calls.

Many fellow enthusiasts have supported our research. I am particularly indebted to Howard Jacobson for writing *The Mighty Walzer*, hands down the finest fusion of literature and table tennis. The United States is all the poorer because this book has not been published here. Our project has been helped exponentially by Andy Spade, Judah Friedlander, Biba Golic and all at Killerspin, Thomas Nguyen and all at Joola, Dan Rollman of URDB.org, Raymond Roker and URB, A. J. Jacobs, Jonathan Safran Foer, Will Shortz, Harry Evans, Rob Stone and all at Cornerstone/FADER whose passion for the game makes them a role model for American youth, Joshua Foer, Ross Martin, Alex Grossman, Courtney Holt, David Katznelson, Josh Kun, Dana Ferine, the inimitable Paul Holdengraber and all at the New York Public Library, and Chris Isenberg, Kimou Meyer, and the No Mas team.

Above all, I am indebted to my entire family. The Krolls, especially Lynn and Jules, Celia Dollar, Simmy and Eric Kirsch, Jamie Glassman, a frustratingly competent paddler and perfect friend, and all the Bennetts: Nigel and Amy. Most important, my lovely mum and dad. I live above a table tennis club in New York City so I know my children are guaranteed to love the game as I did as a kid (though with a mite more class). Samson, Ber, and Zion: may your loop drives always land where you want them to in life. Head and shoulders above everyone, my wife, Vanessa—you are a beautiful woman. There is not a day that goes by that I am unaware of your beauty, intelligence, and understanding. If I still played the game, you would always be my doubles partner, even though we both know the world is a better place because I retired at age eleven.

Eli Horowitz:

On the table in our basement on Loosestrife Court, my father and brother taught me the value of constant defeat; I lost, fell, and got back up and lost again, and they both smiled all the while. My mother tolerated the wreckage we left behind, and instilled in me a love of excessive research.

Simon Huynh, Joshuah Bearman, Nick Hornby, Starlee Kine, Davy Rothbart, and Jesse Aaron Cohen all took this book seriously when there was no real reason to do so; their vital contributions have furthered the advance of truth, ping pong, and friendship—and what else is there?

My collaborators at McSweeney's first taught me how a thought becomes a book, and then restored my faith in ping pong as a language of fellowship.

Roger Bennett willed this book into existence, never wavering in his belief that this story needed to be told and never allowing me to lose faith. He is a scholar and a friend.

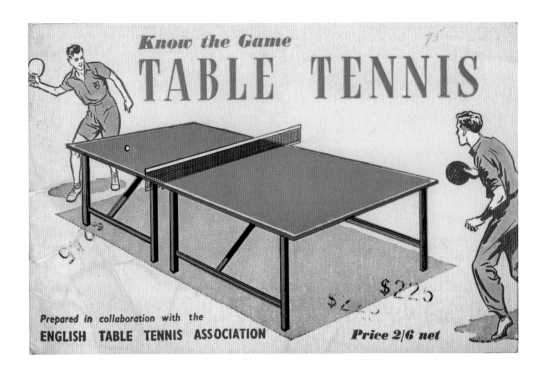

IMMERSE YOURSELF

If reading this book has ignited, reignited, or dangerously inflamed your passion for the game, we could not be more proud. This book is intended as nothing more than a spark, a lantern lighting the path toward a jungle of ping pong enlightenment. The wonderful resources below are some of the pleasures that await you.

USATT is the national organizing body for table tennis in the United States. Founded in 1933, it serves the table tennis community across the country, networking more than 285 clubs, some of which Will Shortz has not even visited yet. The USATT oversees a wide variety of membership services, organizes the national teams, and supervises the rules of the game. Anyone who is interested in the sport will find www.usatt.org to be a great starting point. There is no finer institution in this country.

Tim Boggan's "History of American Table Tennis," hosted on the USATT website, is an invaluable archive for any curious fan. Boggan's essays capture the highs, lows, heroes, and humor of our civilization's first relevant (i.e., pong-present) century. Meticulous and insightful, witty and wise, Boggan is an inspiration and our idol.

The museum of the **International Table Tennis Federation (ITTF)** is located in the depths of Switzerland, but selections from its extensive collection can be viewed online at www.ittf.com/museum. Curator Chuck Hoey has masterfully assembled slide shows capturing the faces and ephemera of the world's greatest game and waged a one-man crusade to preserve its history.

North American Table Tennis, www.natabletennis.com, advances the sport all over the world through application consulting, business development management, event management (including the North American Tour), product development (the iPong Table Tennis Training Buddy is a particular favorite of ours), and distributing the mighty JOOLA brand. The entire management team emerged from the sport, and their passion shines through.

Perhaps the most important site on the entire Internet is **Larry Hodges's collection of photos of celebrities playing table tennis**. With more than 1,038 images at press time, Hodges's trove ranges from Yasser Arafat to Steve Zahn, with plenty of Humphrey Bogart and Sean Connery along the way. Mr. Ed, Richie Rich, 50 Cent—virtually every great icon of our culture makes an appearance in Hodges's exhaustive archive.

Stanislaw Schmidt and his collection of 1,128 different ping pong ball designs carried us through many dark moments. We continue to visit **www.tischtennisbaelle .org** whenever we need a little boost of pure energy. And we discover a new favorite each time.

The proud tradition of hardbat is celebrated by Scott Gordon and his passionate team at **www.hardbat.com**, particularly via their carefully curated footage of classic matches. Another remarkable set of game highlights and ping pong retrospectives can be found at **www.tabletennisvideos.net**.

SPiN New York has brought 13,000 square feet of table tennis majesty straight to the heart of Manhattan. We admire what the club's owners have done to promote the sport, melding style and substance, and urge everyone to stop by and experience ping pong at its most luxurious.

PHOTOGRAPH CREDITS

x   Courtesy of Joola

xii-xiii   Photograph by Arthur Rothstein, courtesy of the Library of Congress

2   Courtesy of the ITTF Museum

5   Courtesy of the ITTF Museum

6   Courtesy of the ITTF Museum

7   Courtesy of the ITTF Museum

11   Photograph by Francis Stewart, courtesy of the Bancroft Library, University of California, Berkeley

18-19   Courtesy of PF Bentley

23   Courtesy of the ITTF Museum

24-25   Photograph by John C. Hemment, courtesy of the Denver Public Library Western Collection

26   Photographs by Stas Kulesh

27   Photograph by Sean Hawkey

28   Photograph by Ben Clarke

29   Photograph by Anne Gunnison, with thanks to Jesse Russell

30   Photograph by Malcolm Anderson

66   Courtesy of the ITTF Museum

68   Courtesy of the ITTF Museum

69   Courtesy of the ITTF Museum

71   Courtesy of the Alabama Department of Archives and History

74   Courtesy of the ITTF Museum

77   Courtesy of the ITTF Museum

78   Courtesy of the ITTF Museum

104-105	Courtesy of Dana and Winnie Ferine
109	Courtesy of Roger Bennett
110	Courtesy of Killerspin
126	Courtesy of the ITTF Museum
127	Courtesy of the ITTF Museum
128	Courtesy of the ITTF Museum
128	Photograph by Malcolm Anderson
135	Courtesy of Össur
136-137	Courtesy of TOSY Robotics JSC
139	Courtesy of the ITTF Museum
158	Photograph by Malcolm Anderson
163	Photographs by Malcolm Anderson
180	Painting by Niklas Nenzén
188	Courtesy of the ITTF Museum
198	Courtesy of Dunlop, with thanks to Ben Fell
200	Photograph by Malcolm Anderson
202	Courtesy of Jack Spade, with thanks to Johanna Saum
202	Courtesy of Roger Bennett, with thanks to Partners & Spade
206	Courtesy of Roy Arad
218	Courtesy of Brookhaven National Laboratory
220	Courtesy of Brookhaven National Laboratory
223	Courtesy of Ralph H. Baer Papers, National Museum of American History
227	Fliers for Puppy Pong, QuadraPong, and Barrel-Pong © 1972 by Atari Interactive, Inc. All rights reserved.
229	Courtesy of Florian Mueller
231	Courtesy of Nyehaus, New York and Cumulus Studios

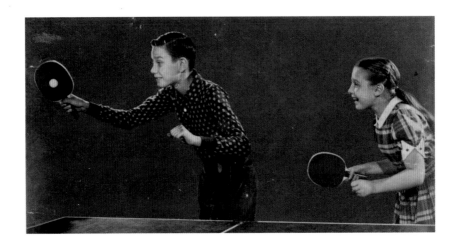

ABOUT THE CONTRIBUTORS

Will Shortz is the crossword editor at the *New York Times* and puzzle master for NPR's *Weekend Edition Sunday*. He plays table tennis on average six times a week and dreams of someday becoming national champion for his age group.

Davy Rothbart is the author of the national bestseller *Found*, and creator of the magazine of the same name. A contributor to public radio's *This American Life*, he is also the author of the story collection *The Lone Surfer of Montana, Kansas*. He lives in Ann Arbor, Michigan.

Starlee Kine is a writer and a frequent contributor to *This American Life*.She lives in New York City and Wallingford, Connecticut.

Howard Jacobson was born in Manchester in 1942. He represented Lancashire in ping pong from 1956 to 1957. He attended Downing College, Cambridge, from 1961 to 1964. He represented Cambridge when Cambridge beat Oxford in 1962. Jacobson lectured on English literature at Sydney University, Selwyn College, Cambridge, and Wolverhampton Polytechnic from 1967 to 1979. Then he became a full-time novelist and critic. He is the author of, among other works, *Coming from Behind, Roots Schmoots, The Mighty*

Walzer (widely regarded as the greatest novel about ping pong ever written), *Kalooki Nights*, and *The Act of Love*. He now makes television documentaries and writes a weekly column for the *Independent*.

Nick Hornby is the author of six novels, most recently *Juliet, Naked*. His screenplay for *An Education* was recently nominated for an Academy Award.

Jonathan Safran Foer is the author of the novels *Everything Is Illuminated* and *Extremely Loud and Incredibly Close*, and the nonfiction book *Eating Animals*.

Harold Evans, former editor of the *Sunday Times* and *The Times of London*, and later president of Random House, is the author of a memoir *My Paper Chase* published by Little, Brown and Company.

Jesse Aaron Cohen lives in Brooklyn. He works as an archivist at the YIVO Institute for Jewish Research and also creates music with Tanlines and Professor Murder.

ABOUT THE AUTHORS

Roger Bennett is the creator of *Bar Mitzvah Disco, Camp Camp, And You Shall Know Us by the Trail of Our Vinyl,* and *ESPN's World Cup Companion*. He has written about sports, music, and culture for the *New York Times, ESPN: The Magazine*, and *Time*, among others. He lives in New York, and ping pong brings out his violent side.

Eli Horowitz designs and edits books for McSweeney's. After a childhood spent consistently losing to his father and brother in their Virginia basement, he captained the third-place intramural ping pong squad at Yale University. He lives in San Francisco.

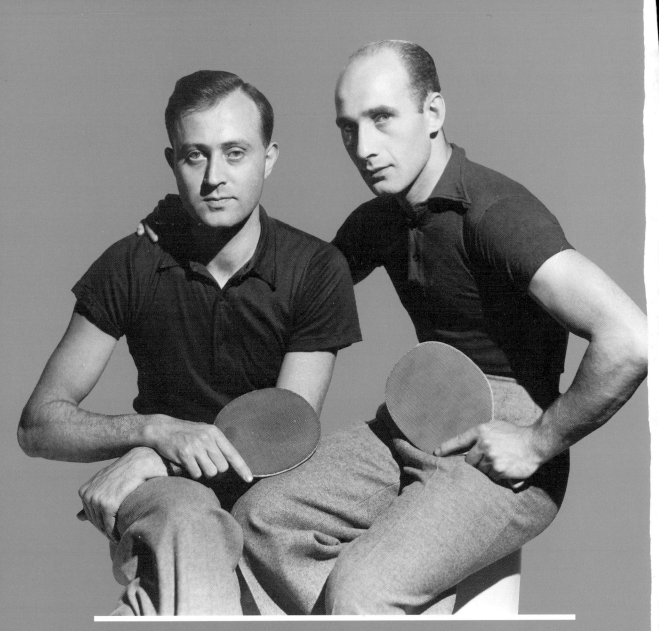

EVERYTHING YOU KNOW IS PONG